English/Chinese Medical Glossary

© **Cross Cultural Health Care Program**
All rights reserved

The Cross Cultural Health Care Program actively protects this copyright.

Chinese Medical Glossary, 2nd Edition
and all other CCHCP publications are not in the public domain.

First Edition 1998, 2nd Edition 2011

No part of this glossary may be reproduced or transmitted in any form or by any means, graphic, electronic, or mechanical, including photocopying, recording, taping or by any information storage or retrieval system, without permission in writing from the Cross Cultural Health Care Program.

The Cross Cultural Health Care Program
4700 42nd Ave SW, Suite 580 | Seattle, WA 98116
(206) 860-0329 | www.xculture.org

English/Chinese Medical Glossary

The Cross Cultural Health Care Program

The Cross Cultural Health Care Program (CCHCP) was established in 1992 in Seattle, Washington with a grant from the W. K. Kellogg Foundation. From the beginning, the organization's goal has been to bridge the gap between underserved communities and services to improve health and well-being.

Now an independent 501(c)(3) nonprofit organization, CCHCP has become the nation's leader in training and resources to overcome language and cultural barriers to health and human services. Each year, CCHCP trains interpreters, providers, and trainers in health and human services, locally and nationally. Widely acknowledged as the creator of the premier 40-hour medical interpreter training program in the nation, CCHCP is a pioneer in many other areas of cultural and linguistic competence. Published resources span a series of nationally respected medical glossaries, ethnic profiles of refugee and immigrant communities, training manuals, videos and research reports. CCHCP builds institutional cultural competence through training, assessment and community-centered research.

For further information, please contact The Cross Cultural Health Care Program, 4700 42nd Ave SW, Suite 580, Seattle, WA 98116, phone 206.860.0329, publications@xculture.org, or **www.xculture.org**.

CCHCP Bilingual Medical Glossaries:

- Amharic
- Arabic
- Bengali
- Bosnian
- Burmese and Karen
- Cambodian Khmer
- Chinese
- English
- French
- Haitian Creole
- Hindi
- Japanese
- Korean
- Lao
- Nepali
- Polish
- Portuguese
- Russian
- Somali
- Spanish
- Tigrigna
- Urdu
- Vietnamese

English/Chinese Medical Glossary

Acknowledgments

We would like to acknowledge CCHCP staff for their contributions to this publication.

Translators:

Primary professional translation by:
   Applied Language Solutions

Assistance from:
The translation was checked by:
   Feng Liao, M.D.
   Emma Ditsworth
   Jaya Lapham

Medical Reviewers

   Marty Babcock, RN, ARNP
   Elizabeth Plotkin, MD
   Thomas Wood, M

English/Chinese Medical Glossary

Preface

This Chinese-English bilingual medical glossary was developed to support the Bridging the Gap medical interpreter training program, which was created to aid the many dedicated individuals around the country who provide interpretation services to limited English-speaking patients in health care settings. In a field where misinterpretation and misunderstanding can be serious and even fatal, finding the "right words" to interpret or translate medical terminology is a tremendous challenge. We hope this glossary helps in that valuable work.

Development of the glossary presented several challenges. First, interpreters, translators, health care providers, public health workers, and staff at CCHCP and CalOptima selected approximately 2,400 words commonly used during the patient-provider encounter. Second, these words were defined appropriately in English in ways they might be used during the patient-provider encounter. And third, these often complex biomedical terms or phrases were translated into both Simplified and Traditional Chinese. During this process we continued to learn more about language, how people use language, and about the process of translation.

The terms and phrases included here range from very technical biomedical terms, such as *hysterectomy*, to less technical but equally challenging terms to translate, such as *shortness of breath*. Although every attempt was made to include the most common terms used during the patient-provider encounter, some may have been left out. This medical glossary is not definitive; it is only intended to provide a foundation in medical terminology.

Each medical term in the glossary is accompanied by an English definition. Each definition captures the meaning and use of a word or phrase in a biomedical context. These definitions were reviewed and edited by medical professionals. Be aware that many of these terms have additional meanings applicable outside of the medical field, and caution should be used with such terms.

For example, in this glossary the word *beat* is defined as "a single contraction of the heart." Outside of medicine, *beat* does not refer to the heart and could be defined as "to strike or hit repeatedly, or a single strike or blow." Selection of the correct terms to use in translations or interpretations is left to the interpreter, but keep in mind the definitions in this glossary focus on the way these terms are used in a biomedical context.

Once defined, the 2,400 words were translated into Chinese. Next, a team of bilingual medical professionals with experience in medical terminology checked each translation and performed back translation to ensure validity.

In every step of this process, the greatest challenge was translating terms out of context. Wolfgang Teubert, a German linguist, clearly explained this barrier in his article Translation and the Dictionary (Institut fur deutsche Sprache - The Tuscan Word Centre Workshop 19th - 21st June 1998);

> Looking at citations from the *Bank of English* (a dictionary), we again demonstrate the difficulty of selecting the proper translation equivalent for the words *sorrow* and *grief*. It seems that the problem with words like these is that they acquire their specific meaning only in connection with the context they occur in. The rules accounting for the selection of a particular word often differ from (English) to (Karen or Burmese). To choose the correct translation equivalent therefore means interpreting the (English) text in which the word in question occurs.

Throughout the glossary are symbols, word phrases, and annotations to help make the translation more transparent; that is, to help the users of this glossary understand how the translator came to choose words or phrases in the translation.

English/Chinese Medical Glossary

Chinese Medical Glossary User Guide

Basic Glossary Structure

Each entry in the glossary has several parts: In order from left to right they are 1) the English biomedical term or phrase, 2) the part-of-speech, 3) an indicator (m) if the word has multiple meanings in English, 4) the English definition, 5) the Traditional translation, 6) the Simplified translation.

Several reference pages have been added at the end of the glossary, containing commonly used words in the categories of The Medical Team, Medical Specialists, Medical Procedures and Exams, Types of Pain, and Medical Equipment.

Excerpt from Medical Glossary:

Term	Definition	Traditional	Simplified
adult (n)	a living organism that has attained full growth or maturity	成年	成年

English Biomedical Term or Phrase

The first column of terms or phrases in the glossary represents our selection of over 2,400 biomedical terms commonly used during the patient-provider encounter. This word list is organized in alphabetical order and grouped by each word's first letter. Terms and phrases are presented in their proper lower-case form except for non-scientific or non-medical names of diseases, such as *Crohn's Disease*.

Several English terms or phrases are accompanied by an additional word or phrase in parentheses "( )". These additional words give the English word more context to how it is being used in this glossary. For example, the term *glasses* was given the following entry:

glasses (eye-) (n)   a pair of lenses mounted in a light frame, used to correct poor vision or to protect the eyes.

Including "(eye)" into the glossary entry helps specify *eye-glasses* instead of the plural version of glass, which is often defined as "a container used for drinking or consuming a liquid."

To provide additional clarity, some English terms are followed by another word or set of words. Often the provider will use this additional word interchangeably with the first term. For example, in the following entry for *allergy shots*:

allergy shots, immunotherapy (n)
    an injection to prevent an allergic reaction.

Allergy shots, in some instances, can be exchanged with *immunotherapy*. However, *immunotherapy* does not share the same definition as *allergy shots*. The interpreter or translator should be aware of the relationship between these words, but should use caution when substituting the second term for the first in translation or interpretation.

Part-of-Speech

Each term or phrase is assigned a part-of-speech that designates how it should be used in a sentence. The part-of-speech abbreviations are defined as follows:

n	noun
adj	adjective
v	verb
prep	prepositional phrase

Multiple Meanings (m)

As explained in the preface, you will find many words listed that have multiple meanings or usages associated with them. To denote this, several key word entries are marked with "(m)". Our definitions focus on their medical definitions.

English Definition

The English definition expresses the meaning of the term or phrase and how it should be used in a biomedical context. Each definition was designed to retain the specific and often technical meaning of a term or phrase while effectively expressing the meaning of the term or phrase so that it could be understood by the general reader. In order to achieve this, many of the definitions convey a broader meaning of the word then focus this definition, such as in the following definition of *poison*:

poison (n)   a substance that causes injury, illness, or death, esp. by chemical means.

Other definitions are expressed through examples and synonyms. Words *italicized* in the definition are specific Latin classification names for organisms.

Abbreviations Used in the English Definition

e.g.   *exempli gratia*, for example

esp.   especially

i.e.   *id est*, that is

etc.   *et cetera*, and so forth

Chinese Translations

Naturally, in a glossary of this type, it is impossible to include all possible regional variations. Our aim has been to define medical terms so as to give the exact or closest equivalent for the English term, and to list as many synonyms as practical. We feel, with the exception of some highly technical terms, that the definitions are readily understandable anywhere in the Chinese-speaking world. Users of this glossary are encouraged to make annotations of regional translations as they become aware of them.

The glossary translates only the English terms or phrases located in the first column of words. It does not translate the definition of terms or phrases.

We hope this glossary will be helpful while interpreting or translating in the medical field. However, no translation is ever "perfect." We welcome comments about the translations, word list, and publication design. This will help us improve future translations of other language glossaries, and in the end, aid other interpreters and translators.

English/Chinese Medical Glossary - A

Term	Definition	Traditional	Simplified
abdomen (n)	part of body between the chest and legs; the cavity of the human body containing the stomach, intestines, liver, gallbladder, pancreas, spleen, etc.; also called the belly	腹部	腹部
abdominal (adj)	of, or pertaining to the abdomen	腹部的	腹部的
abnormal (adj)	not normal; contrary to the usual structure, position, behavior, or rule	異常的	异常的
abortion (n)	the premature expulsion of a fetus from the uterus, or removal of a fetus not capable of living, developing, or functioning successfully	墮胎	堕胎
abrasion (n)	an area of body surface where skin is removed through some mechanical process	擦傷	擦伤
abrupt (adj)	sudden and unexpected	突然的	突然的
abscess (n)	a localized collection of pus in tissues, organs, or confined spaces	膿腫	脓肿
absorption (n)	the uptake of substances into or across tissues, e. g., skin and intestine	吸收	吸收
abstinence (n)	a refraining from the use of food, stimulants, or sexual intercourse	節制，禁戒	节制，禁戒
abuse (v) (m)	to use wrongly or improperly; to misuse a substance, e.g., alcohol, medicine, or drugs	濫用	滥用

English/Chinese Medical Glossary - A

Term	Definition	Traditional	Simplified
access (n)	a patient's ability to obtain medical care. The ease of access is determined by several components, including the availability of medical services and their acceptability to the patients, the location of facilities, transportation, and hours of operation and cost.	接近	接近
accident (n)	an unexpected event	意外事故	意外事故
accommodation (n) (m)	adjustment, such as that of the eye for various distances	調節	调节
accumulation (n)	the action or process of gathering together; state of being or having collected together	蓄積	蓄积
ache (n)	a dull pain	隱痛	隐痛
ache (v)	to suffer a dull pain	疼痛	疼痛
acid (n)	any substance capable of reacting with and dissolving certain metals to form salts, capable of reacting with bases to form salts, or which has a sour stinging taste	酸性物質	酸性物质
acidity (n)	the quality of being acid or sour; the trait of containing acid (hydrogen ions)	酸性	酸性
acne (n)	an inflammatory disease of the hair roots or sebaceous glands, frequently used alone to designate common acne	座瘡	座疮
acquired immuno-deficiency syndrome (AIDS) (n)	disease due to infection with the human immunodeficiency virus (HIV), see AIDS	愛滋病	艾滋病
action plan (n)	a summary of what is intended to be accomplished	工作計畫	工作计划
activate (v)	to set in motion; to create or organize	活化	活化

English/Chinese Medical Glossary - A

Term	Definition	Traditional	Simplified
active (adj)	1. in motion, moving; 2. functioning or capable of functioning	①活動的；②能動的	①活动的；②能动的
Activities of Daily Living (ADLs)	activities performed as part of a person's daily routine of self-care, such as bathing, dressing, toileting, transferring, and eating	日常生活活動	日常生活活动
acuity (n)	clarity or clearness, especially of vision	〔視力〕敏銳	（視力）敏锐
acupuncture (n)	a traditional Chinese therapeutic technique whereby the body is punctured with fine needles	針灸	针灸
acute (adj)	sharp, poignant; having a short and relatively severe course	急性的	急性的
adam's apple (n)	a large visible portion of the larynx located in front of the throat	喉結	喉结
adaptation (n)	the adjustment of an organism to its environment	適應性調節	适应性调节
addiction (n)	the state of being dependent on a habit, especially strong dependence on a drug	癮	瘾
adequate (adj)	satisfactory in quantity or quality; sufficient	足夠的	足够的
adhesion (n)	the joining of two parts or surfaces, such as the joining of two opposing faces of a wound	黏結	黏结
admit (v) (m)	to permit to enter; to have room for	允許進入，容納	允许进入，容纳
adolescent (n)	an individual between puberty and adulthood, mainly in the teenage years	青春期	青春期
adrenal gland (n)	one of two glands located above each kidney that secretes hormones	腎上腺	肾上腺
adult (n)	a living organism that has attained full growth or maturity	成年	成年

English/Chinese Medical Glossary - A

Term	Definition	Traditional	Simplified
Adult Day Center (ADC)	a center that provides a wide range of services for adults who need a protected environment and care from trained staff	成人日間照護中心	成人日间照顾中心
Adult Day Health Center (ADHC) (n)	ADHC provides an individualized treatment plan, nursing and personal care, restorative therapies (physical, occupational, and speech), maintenance therapy, psychological counseling, and nutritional counseling	成人日間健康照護中心	成人日间健康照护中心
Adult Day Treatment Center (ADTC) (n)	a center that specializes in the treatment of people with psychological problems, including dementia, on a short-term basis	成人日間治療中心	成人日间治疗中心
Adult Preventive Services (n)	services to protect adults from getting sick	成人預防服務	成人预防服务
adulthood (adj)	fully developed and mature	成年期的	成年期的
advanced directive (n)	a legal document created by an individual stating his/her wishes; this document may be used to guide medical care during periods when the individual cannot make decisions for himself/herself	醫療治療指示	医疗治疗指示
advanced stage (n)	highly developed or far along in course	晚期，末期	晚期，末期
advanced-registered nurse practitioner (n)	senior ranking nurse capable of prescribing medicines	高級註冊執業護士	高级注册执业护士
adverse effect (n)	undesired result	副作用	副作用
advice (n)	opinion about what could or should be done about a problem	意見	意见
advocate (n)	a person who speaks for others	提倡，代言	提倡，代言
aerobic (adj)	requiring oxygen	需氧的	需氧的

English/Chinese Medical Glossary - A

Term	Definition	Traditional	Simplified
aerobic exercise (n)	continuous and vigorous activity, such as running or cycling, that uses oxygen and builds endurance of the heart and lungs	有氧運動	有氧运动
aerosol (n)	a solid or liquid drug carried in a fine mist for inhalation therapy	噴劑	喷剂
affiliate (n)	an organization or person that directly or indirectly, through one or more intermediaries, controls, is controlled by, or is under the control of the contractor and provides services to or receives services from the contractor	附屬機構	附属机构
affinity (n)	a special attraction for a specific element, organ, or structure	親合力	亲合力
afterbirth (n)	placenta and umbilical cord expelled from the uterus after childbirth	胞衣	胞衣
agent (n) (m)	any power, principle, or substance capable of producing an effect, whether physical, chemical, or biological	藥劑	药剂
aggravation (n)	an increase in seriousness or severity; an act or circumstance that intensifies, or makes worse	加重，惡化	加重，恶化
aggression (n)	hostile behavior	攻擊行為	攻击行为
aggressive (adj)	the quality of being inclined to move or act in a violent or hostile manner	攻擊性的	攻击性的
agitation (n)	a state of being upset; disturbance; commotion	躁動	躁动
AIDS (n)	disease due to infection with the human immunodeficiency virus (HIV). AIDS is an acronym for Acquired Immuno-Deficiency Syndrome	愛滋病	艾滋病

English/Chinese Medical Glossary - A

Term	Definition	Traditional	Simplified
ailment (n)	a physical or mental disorder	疾病	疾病
air lift (n)	a system of transporting patients by air when surface routes are blocked	空運	空运
airway (n)	a passage in which air enters the body, e.g., trachea, bronchi, and lungs	呼吸道	呼吸道
airway obstruction (n)	any object or substance that prevents breathing by blocking the passage of air into the lungs	氣道梗阻	气道梗阻
albumin (n)	a type of protein	白蛋白	白蛋白
alcohol (n)	a water soluble molecule; an intoxicating liquor	醇	醇
alcoholic beverage (n)	an intoxicating beverage; spirit	酒精飲料	酒精饮料
Alcoholism (n)	a disorder characterized by excessive alcohol use that causes serious impairment in physical, social or occupational functioning	酒精濫用，酗酒	酒精濫用，酗酒
alert (adj)	attentive and quick to think or act	警覺的	警觉的
alkaline (adj)	relating to or containing an aqueous solution that is bitter, slippery, and characteristically basic in chemical reactions	鹼性	碱性
allergen (n)	a substance that causes an allergy	過敏原	过敏原
allergic (adj)	causing allergy; having an allergy	過敏的	过敏的
allergic reaction (n)	a physical response to an allergen	過敏反應	过敏反应
allergic rhinitis (n)	medical term for hay fever, a condition due to allergy that mimics a chronic cold	過敏性鼻炎	过敏性鼻炎
allergist (n)	a physician specializing in allergies	過敏症專科醫生	过敏症专科医生

English/Chinese Medical Glossary - A

Term	Definition	Traditional	Simplified
allergy (n)	an extreme sensitivity to environmental factors or substances, such as pollens, dust, or foods, that causes a pathological response, such as a rash or difficulty in breathing	過敏症	过敏症
allergy shots, immunotherapy (n)	an injection to prevent an allergic reaction	過敏注射	过敏注射
alpha-fetoprotein test (n)	a test used to detect disease and some tumors in a fetus	甲胎球蛋白檢查	甲胎球蛋白检查
alternate (v)	to change from one to another, sometimes back and forth	輪流	轮流
alternative (n) (m)	something that is available in place of something else	替代物	替代物
Alzheimer's Day Care Resource Centers (ADCRC) (n)	a center specializing in programs for persons with Alzheimer's disease or related dementia	老年癡呆症日間護理中心	老年痴呆症日间护理中心
Alzheimer's Disease (n)	a severe mental disorder marked by progressive decrease in intellectual capabilities	阿爾茨海默病	阿尔茨海默病
ambulance (n)	a vehicle specially equipped to transport the sick or wounded	救護車	救护车
ambulant (adj)	moving or walking about; having the ability to move	能走動的	能走动的
ambulatory care (adj)	any type of health service that is provided on an outpatient basis	門診醫療	门诊医疗
amenorrhea (n)	abnormal suppression or absence of menstruation	停經	停经
American Academy of Ophthalmology (n)	an organization of opthalmologists (eye doctors) dedicated to providing comprehensive eye care	美國眼科醫學會	美国眼科医学会

English/Chinese Medical Glossary - A

Term	Definition	Traditional	Simplified
American Cancer Society (n)	a nationwide community-based voluntary health organization dedicated to eliminating cancer as a major health problem by: preventing cancer, saving lives, and diminishing suffering from cancer, through research, education, advocacy, and service	美國癌症學會	美国癌症学会
amino acid (n)	an organic compound which is the foundation of any of various proteins, and is important for proper body function	氨基酸	氨基酸
amnesia (n)	lack or loss of memory; inability to remember past experiences	遺忘症	遗忘症
amniocentesis (n)	the surgical withdrawal of a sample of fluid from the uterus of a pregnant woman	羊膜穿刺術	羊膜穿刺术
amniotic fluid (n)	the fluid surrounding a fetus	羊膜水	羊膜水
amphetamine (n)	a drug used to excite the central nervous system	安非他命，苯丙胺	苯丙胺
ampoule (n)	a small glass or plastic container capable of being sealed to protect its contents from contamination	安瓿	安瓿
amputation (n)	the act or process of removing a body part, esp. an extremity including a finger, toe, hand, arm, foot, or leg	截肢	截肢
anaerobic (adj)	lacking molecular oxygen; growing, living, or occurring in the absence of molecular oxygen	厭氧的	厌氧的
analgesic (n)	a medication that reduces or eliminates pain	止痛劑	止痛剂
analysis (n)	an examination of a complex issue or substance by looking at the parts and their relations	分析	分析

English/Chinese Medical Glossary - A

Term	Definition	Traditional	Simplified
anaphylaxis (n)	a high sensitivity to foreign substances	超敏性反應	超敏性反应
anatomical (adj)	pertaining to anatomy, or to the structure of the organism	解剖學的	解剖学的
anatomy (n)	any physical structure of the human body including organs, bone, muscle, and nerves	解剖學	解剖学
anemia (n)	a condition of an abnormally low number of red blood cells	貧血	贫血
anemic (adj)	suffering from anemia	貧血的	贫血的
anesthesia (n)	1. loss of feeling or sensation; 2. induced loss of pain, to permit surgery or other painful procedures	麻醉	麻醉
anesthesiologist (n)	a physician who studies and administers anesthetics	麻醉學家	麻醉学家
anesthesiology (n)	the medical study and application of anesthetics	麻醉學	麻醉学
anesthetic (adj)	a drug or agent that is used to abolish the sensation of pain	麻醉的	麻醉的
anesthetist (n)	a person, usually a physician, trained to administer anesthetics	麻醉師	麻醉师
anesthetize (v)	to cause someone total or partial loss of sensation	使麻醉	使麻醉
aneurysm (n)	a sac formed in the wall of an artery, a vein, or the heart	動脈瘤	动脉瘤
angina (n)	a severe constricting pain in the chest	心絞痛	心绞痛
angina pectoris (n)	a severe constricting pain in the chest, often extending from the chest to the left shoulder and down the arm, caused usually by heart disease	心絞痛	心绞痛
angiogram (n)	an image of blood vessels created by injecting x-ray-visible fluid into the blood	血管造影片	血管造影片
angiography (n)	imaging of blood vessels following injection with a contrast material (visible by x-ray)	血管造影術	血管造影术

English/Chinese Medical Glossary - A

Term	Definition	Traditional	Simplified
anguish (n)	an agonizing physical or mental pain; torment	極度痛苦	极度痛苦
ankle (n)	the joint, consisting of the bones and related structure, that connects the foot to the leg	踝，踝關節	踝，踝关节
anomaly (n)	marked deviation from the normal standard	反常	反常
anorexia (n) (m)	lack or loss of the appetite for food	厭食症	厌食症
antacid (n)	a substance that counteracts or neutralizes acidity, usually of the stomach	解酸劑	解酸剂
antagonist (n)	a drug that counteracts or neutralizes another drug	對抗劑	对抗剂
antecedent (n)	an event or thing existing or occurring previously	先例	先例
anterograde (n)	moving or extending forward; also called antegrade	順行	顺行
antibiotic (n)	a drug used to treat bacterial infections	抗生素	抗生素
anuresis (n)	the inability to urinate	無尿症	无尿症
anus (n)	the distal or terminal opening of the digestive system, through which feces are discharged	肛門	肛门
anvil (n)	incus; small bone of the ear	砧骨	砧骨
anxiety (n)	a state of uneasiness and distress about something that is happening or may happen in the future, worry	焦慮	焦虑
anxiety disorder (n)	an illness with the following key symptoms: nervousness, apprehension, fear, worries	焦慮症	焦虑症
anxious (n)	worried and distressed about some uncertain event or matter; uneasy	不安的，焦慮的	不安的，焦虑的
aorta (n)	the largest artery in the human body; it carries blood away from the heart to the limbs	主動脈	主动脉

English/Chinese Medical Glossary - A

Term	Definition	Traditional	Simplified
apathy (n)	lack of feeling or emotion; indifference	淡漠	淡漠
aphasia (n)	defect or loss of the power of expression by speech, writing, or signs, or of comprehending spoken or written language, due to injury or disease of the brain	失語症	失语症
aplastic anemia (n)	bone marrow disorder characterized by a reduction in the number of red blood cells, white blood cells, and platelets	再生障礙性貧血	再生障碍性贫血
apnea (n)	absence of breathing	呼吸暫停	呼吸暂停
appeal (v)	a formal request by a patient or provider for reconsideration of a decision, such as a utilization review recommendation, a benefit payment or an administrative action, with the goal of finding a mutually acceptable solution	要求	要求
appendectomy (n)	the surgical removal of the appendix	蘭尾切除術	阑尾切除术
appendicitis (n)	inflammation of the appendix	蘭尾炎	阑尾炎
appendix (n)	a narrow worm-like appendage attached to the beginning of the large intestine	蘭尾	阑尾
appetite (n)	a desire for food or drink	食欲	食欲
application (n) (m)	the act of bringing something into nearness or contact with another substance; the act of putting something to special use	敷貼，實施	敷贴，实施
applicator (n)	an instrument used to apply a medication or substance	敷料器	敷料器
appointment (n)	an arrangement to do something or meet someone at a particular time and place	約定	约定
aqueous (adj)	watery; prepared with water	水性的	水性的

English/Chinese Medical Glossary - A

Term	Definition	Traditional	Simplified
aqueous humor (n)	a clear bodily fluid found in the eye	〔眼內〕水狀液	（眼內）水狀液
arch (n)	a curved portion of the bottom of the foot	足弓	足弓
arch support or insert (n)	an item used usually in a shoe to support the arch on the bottom of the foot	護弓墊	护弓垫
arm (n)	an upper limb of the human body connecting the hand and wrist to the shoulder	臂	臂
armpit (n)	the hollow under the arm at the shoulder	腋窩	腋窝
arrhythmia (n)	any variation from the normal rhythm of the heart beat	心律失常	心律失常
arterial (adj)	pertaining to an artery or to the arteries	動脈的	动脉的
arteriography (n)	an x-ray of arteries after injection of material into the blood stream	動脈搏描記法，動脈造影術	动脉搏描记法，动脉造影术
arteriosclerosis (n)	a chronic disease in which thickening and hardening of arterial walls makes blood circulation difficult	小動脈硬化	小动脉硬化
artery (n)	any of a branching system of tubes that carry blood away from the heart	動脈	动脉
artery wall (n)	the inner surface that makes an artery	動脈壁	动脉壁
arthralgia (n)	pain in a joint	關節痛	关节痛
arthritis (n)	inflammation of a joint or joints	關節炎	关节炎
arthrogram (n)	an image of a joint after the injection of x-ray-visible fluid	關節造影片	关节造影片
arthrosclerosis (n)	stiffness of the joints, especially in the aged	關節硬化	关节硬化
arthroscopy (n)	a procedure that allows direct examination of a joint using a small camera	關節內窺鏡檢查	关节内窥镜检查
articular (adj)	of, or pertaining to a joint	關節的	关节的

English/Chinese Medical Glossary - A

Term	Definition	Traditional	Simplified
articular capsulitis (n)	inflammation of a joint capsule, such as the shoulder, knee, or elbow	關節囊炎	关节囊炎
articulation (n) (m)	1. the act or process of speaking; 2. the method or manner of joining; 3. a joint between two bones or between movable parts	①發音；②接合；③（骨頭）的關節	①发音；②接合；③（骨头）的关节
artificial (adj)	not natural	人造的	人造的
artificial insemination (n)	the introduction of semen into the female reproductive organs without sexual contact	人工受孕	人工受孕
ascending colon (n)	the first section of the large intestine	上行結腸	上行结肠
asepsis (n)	absence of infection	無菌	无菌
aseptic (adj)	of, or pertaining to the state of being free of pathogenic organisms	無菌的	无菌的
aspiration (n)	1. the act of inhaling; 2. withdrawal of fluid from the body	①吸入；②抽出液體	①吸入；②抽出液体
aspirator (n)	an instrument used to remove fluid from a cavity	抽吸器	抽吸器
assay (n)	1. a procedure to study a substance, esp. a drug; 2. a substance to be studied; 3. the result of such study	①化驗；②被分析物；③化驗結果	①化验；②被分析物；③化验结果
assist (v)	to give support or aid	協助	协助
association (n) (m)	1. the act of joining in a relationship; 2. the act of connecting or joining together; 3. the act of connecting in the mind or imagination	①締合；②聯合；③聯想	①缔合；②联合；③联想
asthma (n)	a chronic respiratory disease, often arising from allergies, and accompanied by labored breathing, chest constriction, and coughing	哮踹	哮踹
asthmatic (adj)	pertaining to a person with or who suffers from asthma	哮踹的	哮踹的

English/Chinese Medical Glossary - A

Term	Definition	Traditional	Simplified
astigmatism (n)	faulty vision caused by defects in the lens of the eye	散光	散光
astringent (adj)	topical drug that causes contraction, often found in lotion	收斂的	收敛的
asymptomatic (adj)	showing or causing no symptoms	無症狀的	无症状的
ataxia (n)	loss or lack of muscular coordination	共濟失調	共济失调
atelectasis (n)	lack of gas from part or the whole of the lungs	（肺）膨脹不全	（肺）膨胀不全
atheroma (n)	1. fat deposits on the walls of medium and large arteries; 2. a sebaceous cyst	①動脈粥樣化；②粉瘤	①动脉粥样化；②粉瘤
atherosclerosis (n)	see *arteriosclerosis*	動脈硬化	动脉硬化
athetosis (n)	a condition of endless slow involuntary movements	手足徐動症	手足徐动症
athlete's foot, tinea pedis (n)	a contagious skin infection caused by fungi, usually affecting the feet and sometimes the hands, and causing itching, blistering, cracking, and scaling	足癬	足癣
atrium (n) (m)	1. a chamber; 2. chamber acting as an entrance to another structure or organ; 3. a specific section of the heart	①心房；②前房	①心房；②前房
atrophy (n)	a wasting away; a reduction in size of a cell, tissue, organ, or part	萎縮	萎缩
attack (v)	to use violent force	用力，攻擊	用力，攻击
attending physician (n)	a physician primarily in charge of a patient's care in the hospital and who oversees the medical practice of residents	主治醫生	主治医生
Attention Deficit/Hyperactive Disorder (n)	biological disorder that causes the suffer to be easily distracted, impulsive, and restless, it occurs more frequently in boys than in girls	注意力缺失/過動症	注意力缺失/过动症

English/Chinese Medical Glossary - A

Term	Definition	Traditional	Simplified
atypical (adj)	irregular; not conformable to the type	非典型的	非典型的
audiologist (n)	a person who studies hearing defects and their treatment	聽力學家	听力学家
auditory (adj)	pertaining to the sense of hearing	聽覺的	听觉的
auditory nerve (n)	a nerve that sends signals to the brain, enabling someone to hear	聽神經	听神经
aural (adj)	pertaining to, or perceived by the ear	耳的	耳的
auricle (n)	the external portion of the ear	耳廓	耳廓
auricular (adj)	relating to the ear	心耳的	心耳的
auscultation (n)	the act of listening for sounds within the body with a stethoscope, chiefly for determining the condition of the lungs, heart, and abdomen	聽診	听诊
authority (n)	persons in command, specifically a governmental agency or corporation to administer a revenue-producing public enterprise	當局	当局
autoimmune (adj)	related to or caused by antibodies	自身免疫的	自身免疫的
autopsy (n)	examination of a dead body to determine cause of death	屍體解剖	尸体解剖
autotransfusion (n)	a method of returning blood back into the body	自體輸血	自体输血
axilla (n)	armpit, underarm	腋窩	腋窝

Notes

English/Chinese Medical Glossary - A

English/Chinese Medical Glossary - B

baby bottle (n)	a bottle containing baby formula or another type of liquid to be consumed by a baby	嬰兒奶瓶	婴儿奶瓶
baby formula (n)	a liquid food containing required nutrients for a newborn baby	嬰兒奶粉	婴儿奶粉
baby teeth (n)	the first set of teeth to grow in a baby	乳牙	乳牙
back (n) (m)	the rear area of the human from the neck to the waist	背	背
back of knee (n)	the region on the backside of the knee	膝彎	膝弯
back of neck, nape (n)	the rear area of the neck	頸背	颈背
backache (n)	a pain or discomfort in the region of the back or spine	背痛	背痛
backbone (n)	the vertebrate spine or spinal column; the major support of the back in a human	脊骨	脊骨
background (n)	1. the circumstances and events surrounding or leading up to something; 2. a person's total experience, education, and knowledge	背景	背景
bacteria (n)	see *bacterium*	細菌	细菌
bacterial infection (n)	a specific pathology caused by bacteria, causing injury to tissue	細菌感染	细菌感染
bactericide (n)	an agent that destroys bacteria	殺菌劑	杀菌剂
bacteriological (adj)	pertaining to the study of bacteria	細菌學家	细菌学家
bacteriostatic (adj)	inhibiting the growth or multiplication of bacteria	抑菌的	抑菌的
bacterium (n)	one of a group of very small organisms that can be free-living or parasites, and have a wide range of pathogenic properties; singular of bacteria	細菌	细菌
bad breath (n)	an unpleasant smell originating from the mouth, caused by some foods and not cleaning the teeth	口臭	口臭
bad taste (n)	an unpleasant flavor	異味	异味

English/Chinese Medical Glossary - B

balance (n)	1. the act of bringing or keeping equal; 2. satisfying proportion or harmony; 3. the ability to stand without falling; 4. the amount owed after a partial settlement, whatever is left over, remainder	平衡	平衡
bald (adj)	the condition of not having hair, esp. on the head	禿的	禿的
ball of foot (n)	the padded portion of the sole of the foot closest to the toes	蹠骨球	跖骨球
bandage (n)	a strip of fabric or other material used as a protective covering for a wound or other injury	繃帶	绷带
barium enema (n)	the use of barium to help obtain an x-ray image of the colon	鋇劑灌腸	钡剂灌肠
barrier (n)	an obstruction	阻礙	阻礙
basal (adj)	pertaining to or situated near a base, esp. basal temperature used in family planning	基底的	基底的
base (n) (m)	in chemistry, the non-acid part of a salt; a substance that combines with acids to form salts	基底	基底
bathtub (n)	a tub for bathing, esp. one permanently installed in a bathroom	浴缸	浴缸
battered child (n)	a child that has experienced physical or mental abuse	受虐待的孩子	受虐待的孩子
beat (n) (m)	a single contraction of the heart	搏動	搏动
bed of the nail (n)	the part of the finger or toe where a nail begins to grow	甲床	甲床
bedbug (n)	a wingless, bloodsucking insect that has a flat, reddish body and a disagreeable odor and that often infests human dwellings	臭蟲	臭虫
bedpan (n)	a metal, glass, or plastic container for receiving human bodily waste	便盆	便盆

English/Chinese Medical Glossary - B

bedridden (n)	the condition of not being able to leave one's bed because of disease, injury, or illness	臥床不起	卧床不起
bedsore (n)	a skin ulcer caused by laying in bed for an extended period of time	褥瘡	褥疮
bedwetting (n)	involuntary discharge of urine while sleeping	遺尿症	遗尿症
behavioral health care (n)	therapy aimed at modification of behavior	行為醫學照護	行为医学照护
belch (v)	to expel gas noisily from the stomach through the mouth	打嗝	打嗝
belief (n)	the mental act, condition, or habit of placing trust or confidence in a person or thing	相信	相信
belief system (n)	the organization and framework of a person or group's beliefs	信念系統	信念系统
Bell's Palsy (n)	a condition/disease characterized by a sudden loss of sensation and movement of the face, thought to be caused by a virus	貝爾氏麻痺	贝尔氏麻痹
belly (n)	the stomach; the abdomen	腹	腹
belly button (n)	the navel; the scar on the abdomen left after the umbilical cord is removed	臍	脐
belt (n)	a strap of leather or cloth worn around the waist and used to support clothing	腰帶	腰带
bend over (v)	to assume a position where the body is leaning over at the waist; to bow	彎腰	弯腰
beneficiary (n)	any person eligible to receive services agreed upon in a contract	受益人	受益人
benefit package (n)	services offered by an insurer to a group of individuals under the terms of a contract	福利計劃	福利计划
benign (adj)	not malignant; favorable for recovery	良性	良性

English/Chinese Medical Glossary - B

Beri Beri (n)	a disease caused by a deficiency or lack of thiamine, an essential nutrient, and that produces numerous problems including neurological disorders	腳氣病	脚气病
beverage (n)	any liquid made for drinking	飲料	饮料
bewitched (n)	the condition of being placed under someone's power by or as if by magic; cast under a spell	著魔	着魔
bifocal glasses (n)	glasses capable of assisting someone's vision at two different distances, usually for reading and for looking at distant objects	雙焦點眼鏡	双焦点眼镜
big toe (n)	the largest toe on the foot	大腳趾	大脚趾
bike helmet (n)	protective gear for the head worn as a hat	自行車頭盔	自行车头盔
bilateral (adj)	having two sides, or pertaining to both sides	兩側的	两侧的
bile (n)	a bitter, alkaline, brownish-yellow or greenish-yellow liquid that is secreted by the liver, stored in the gall bladder, and discharged into the small intestines; it aids in digestion, chiefly by dissolving fats	膽汁	胆汁
bile duct (n)	any of the passages in the liver that move bile from the liver and gallbladder to the intestines	膽管	胆管
biliary (adj)	pertaining to the bile, to the bile ducts, or to the gallbladder	膽汁的	胆汁的
bilirubin (n)	the orange or yellow substance in bile	膽紅素	胆红素
bill (n)	an itemized list or statement of fees or charges	帳單	帐单
biological (adj)	pertaining to biology	生物學的	生物学的
biological clock (n)	a biological mechanism responsible for the time-dependent aspects of a living organism	生物鐘	生物钟

English/Chinese Medical Glossary - B

biology (n)	the science of living organisms and life processes, including the study of structure, function, growth, origin, evolution, and distribution of living organisms	生物學	生物学
biopsy (n)	the removal and examination, usually microscopic, of tissue from the living body, performed to establish precise diagnosis	活組織檢查	活组织检查
birth (n)	the beginning of existence; fact of being born; the act of bearing young; the passage of a child from the uterus	分娩	分娩
birth canal (n)	the canal through which the baby passes in birth	產道	产道
birth certificate (n)	an official document recording the facts of birth, including date, time, and place, and names of the newborn's parents	出生證	出生证
birth control (pill) (n)	a pill for the prevention of unwanted pregnancy	避孕(藥)	避孕(药)
birth date (n)	the day of one's birth, according to the calendar	出生日期	出生日期
birth defect (n)	any of numerous problems found with a baby at birth	先天缺損	先天缺损
birth mark (n)	a mole or blemish present on the body from birth	胎記	胎记
bite (v)	to cut, grip, or tear with or as if with the teeth	咬傷	咬伤
blackhead (n)	a plug of dried fatty matter capped with blackened dust and skin that clogs a pore of the skin	黑頭粉刺	黑头粉刺
bladder (n)	a sac that stores fluid, such as urine or bile	膀胱	膀胱
bleed (v)	to lose blood	出血	出血
bleeding nose (n)	to lose or emit blood from the nose	流鼻血	流鼻血
blemish (n)	a coloring or defect of the skin caused usually by a bruise, pimple, or scar	瑕疵	瑕疵

English/Chinese Medical Glossary - B

blind (adj)	being without sight; sightless	瞎的	瞎的
blind spot (n)	a region of a person's visual field where he or she cannot see	盲點	盲点
blink (v)	to close and open the eyes	眨眼	眨眼
blister (n)	a thin, rounded swelling of the skin, containing watery matter, caused by burning or irritation	水泡	水泡
bloated (adj)	a condition, feeling or sensation of being filled or swollen with water or air	腹脹	腹胀
block (n)	an obstruction or stoppage	阻斷	阻断
blockage (n)	an obstruction or stoppage, esp. of a blood vessel or intestine	阻滯	阻滞
blood (n)	the fluid circulated by the heart through the vascular system that carries oxygen and nutrients throughout the body and transports waste materials to organs that will remove the waste	血液	血液
blood bank (n)	a place where whole blood is typed, processed, and stored for future use in transfusion	血庫	血库
blood cell (n)	a red or white blood cell capable of transporting waste and oxygen or assisting in fighting a disease	血細胞	血细胞
blood clot (n)	a solid mass of blood	血塊	血块
blood count (n)	the number of red and white blood cells in a specific volume of blood	血細胞計數	血细胞计数
blood culture (n)	a procedure of growing or developing blood cells outside of the body	血培養	血培养
blood pressure (n)	the pressure of the blood within the arteries, primarily maintained by the heart	血壓	血压
blood pressure cuff (n)	an instrument used to measure blood pressure	血壓表袖套	血压表袖套
blood relative (n)	a person who is related by birth rather than by marriage	血親	血亲
blood serum (n)	the liquid part of blood	血清	血清

English/Chinese Medical Glossary - B

blood sugar level (n)	the concentration of sugar (glucose) in the blood. It is usually measured in milligrams per deciliter (mg/dl)	血糖數值	血糖数值
blood sugar, glucose (n)	the amount of glucose and other sugars in the blood	血糖	血糖
blood test (n)	an examination of a blood sample	驗血	验血
blood thinner (n)	a drug that helps prevent blood clots	血液抗凝劑	血液抗凝剂
blood transfusion (n)	the introduction of whole blood or blood component directly into the blood stream	輸血	输血
blood type (n)	a system that categorizes blood according to specific chemical attributes	血型	血型
blood vessel (n)	an elastic, tubular canal, such as an artery, vein, or capillary, through which blood circulates	血管	血管
bloody stool (n)	feces that is red in color and contains red blood cells	血便	血便
blow (v) (m)	to expel air from the mouth	吹氣	吹气
blurred vision (n)	vision that is hazy in outline or appearance; dim	視線模糊	视线模糊
board certified (n)	refers to a physician who has passed an examination given by a medical specialty board and who has been certified as a specialist in that medical area	認證醫生	认证医生
board eligible (n)	refers to a physician who is eligible to take the specialty board examination by virtue of having graduated from an approved medical school, completed a specific type and length of training, and practiced for a specified amount of time	醫師資格證	医师资格证
Board of Directors (n)	a group of people who make policy decisions for an organization	董事會	董事会

English/Chinese Medical Glossary - B

body (n)	a group of organs and tissues working together to perform human functions; these functions include: the nervous system, circulatory system, respiratory system, skeletal and muscular system, digestive system, and the reproductive system	身體	身体
body cell (n)	the basic unit or building block of all living matter that makes up organs that work together to perform major functions	體細胞	体细胞
boil, carbuncle (n)	a painful, localized pus-filled swelling of the skin caused by infection	癰	痈
bone (n)	the dense, semi-rigid, porous, calcified connective tissue of the skeleton	骨	骨
bone fracture (n)	a partial or complete break in a bone	骨折	骨折
bone marrow (n)	the soft material that fills bone cavities, consisting, in varying proportions, of fat cells, growing blood cells, supporting connective tissue and numerous blood vessels	骨髓	骨髓
bone marrow transplant (n)	the surgical procedure of transferring bone marrow from one human to another	骨髓移植	骨髓移植
bone scan (n)	a procedure that uses radiation to diagnose bone diseases	骨骼掃描	骨骼扫描
bone socket (n)	the hollow part of a joint that receives the end of a bone	骨臼	骨臼
booster shot (n)	a supplementary dose of a vaccine injected to maintain immunity	強化注射劑量	强化注射剂量
bottle (n)	a container, usually glass, having a narrow neck and a mouth that can be plugged, corked, or capped	瓶子	瓶子

English/Chinese Medical Glossary - B

bottle feeding (n)	a method of feeding a baby with liquid contained in a bottle, usually milk or baby formula	奶瓶哺養	奶瓶哺養
bowel (n)	an intestine, esp. of a human being	腸	肠
bowel incontinence (n)	a condition of being unable to control the evacuation of the bowels	腸失禁	肠失禁
bowel movement (n)	the passing of substances through the intestines	大便	大便
brace (n) (m)	a device that holds or fastens two or more parts together or in place; clamp	支持〔保護〕支架	支持（保護） 支架
brain (n)	a portion of the central nervous system that is responsible for the interpretation of sensory impulses, the coordination and control of bodily activities, and the exercise of emotion and thought	腦	脑
brain damage (n)	injury to the brain that is caused by various conditions, such as head trauma, inadequate oxygen supply, infection, or intracranial hemorrhage, and that may be associated with a behavioral or functional abnormality	腦損傷	脑损伤
break (v) (m)	to crack or split into two or more pieces with sudden or violent force, esp. a bone	折斷	折断
break out (v)	to quickly develop (e.g., a skin rash, epidemic)	暴發	暴发
breast (n)	the human mammary gland	乳房	乳房
breast cancer (n)	a tumor growth in a mammary gland	乳癌	乳癌
breast feed (v)	to feed (a baby) mother's milk from the breast; suckle	哺乳	哺乳
breast mass (n)	a lump found on the breast, which may suggest cancer	乳腺腫塊	乳腺肿块

English/Chinese Medical Glossary - B

breast pump (n)	an instrument that assists the secretion and collection of milk from the breast	吸乳器	吸乳器
breath (n)	the air inhaled and exhaled in respiration	氣息	气息
breathe (v)	to take air in and out of the body	呼吸	呼吸
breathing (n)	the act or process of respiration	呼吸	呼吸
breathing difficulty (n)	having a hard time moving air in and out of the body	呼吸困難	呼吸困难
breathing machine (n)	ventilator; an instrument that assists someone's respiration, ensuring that an adequate amount of oxygen reaches the lungs and that adequate carbon dioxide is removed	呼吸機	呼吸机
breech (n)	buttocks; lower rear portion of the body	臀部	臀部
bridge of nose (n)	the hard upper part of the nose	鼻樑	鼻梁
broken (adj) (m)	of, or pertaining to a bone that has split or cracked into two or more pieces	破裂的	破裂的
bronchial (adj)	pertaining to one or more bronchi	支氣管的	支气管的
bronchiogenic carcinoma (n)	cancer originating in the bronchi	支氣管原癌	支气管原癌
bronchitis (n)	inflammation of one or more bronchi	支氣管炎	支气管炎
bronchopneumonia (n)	inflammation of the lungs, which usually begins in the terminal bronchioles	支氣管肺炎	支气管肺炎
bronchopulmonary (adj)	pertaining to the lungs and their air passages; both bronchial and pulmonary	支氣管肺的	支气管肺的
bronchoscopy (n)	a slender tubular instrument with a small light on the end for inspection of the interior of the bronchi	支氣管鏡檢查	支气管镜检查
bronchospasm (n)	uncontrollable movement of the smooth muscle of the bronchi, as occurs in asthma	支氣管痙攣	支气管痉挛

English/Chinese Medical Glossary - B

bronchus (n)	either of the two air passages (pl. bronchi) beyond the windpipe that provide a way for air to enter the lungs	支氣管	支气管
bruise (n)	an injury in which the skin is not broken; contusion	挫傷，瘀血	挫伤，瘀血
buccal (adj)	pertaining to or directed toward the cheek or mouth	頰的	颊的
buckle up (v)	to fasten two strap or belt ends	繫緊	系紧
bulimia nervosa (n)	an insatiable appetite, often interrupted by periods of anorexia; bulimia is a psychological disorder that can be accompanied by self-induced vomiting	飲食失常	饮食失常
bullet (n)	a spherical or pointed projectile that is fired from a pistol, rifle, or gun	彈	弹
bullet wound (n)	the injury caused by a bullet	槍彈傷	枪弹伤
bunion (n)	a painful, inflamed swelling on the big toe	趾囊炎	趾囊炎
burn (n)	an injury produced by fire, heat, or a heat-producing agent	燒傷	烧伤
burn (v)	to damage or injure by fire, heat, or a heat-producing agent	灼傷	灼伤
burning pain (n)	physical discomfort marked by intense heat	灼痛	灼痛
burning sensation (n)	feeling marked by intense heat	灼覺	灼觉
burp (v)	to belch, esp. after eating	打嗝	打嗝
bursitis (n)	inflammation of a sac-like bodily cavity, esp. one located between the joints or at points of friction between two moving structures	粘液囊炎	粘液囊炎
business office (n)	a location where a person engages in an occupation, work, or trade	辦事處	办事处
bust (n) (m)	the woman's chest; breasts	胸部	胸部
bust (v) (m)	to break open or burst	打碎	打碎

English/Chinese Medical Glossary - B

buttock (n)	either of the two rounded, fleshy parts of the rump or backside of a human	臀部（半邊）	臀部（半边）
bypass (n) (m)	an alternative passage created surgically between two blood vessels, esp. to avoid an obstruction	分路，分流 血管搭橋	分路，分流， 血管搭橋

Notes

English/Chinese Medical Glossary - C

caffeine (n)	a bitter substance found in coffee, tea, and soda, and used as a stimulant or diuretic	咖啡因	咖啡因
calcium deficiency (n)	low levels of calcium in the blood preventing proper functioning of the body; see *deficiency*	缺鈣	缺钙
calcium (n)	a silvery, moderately hard metallic element essential to the proper functioning of the human body, found mostly in bone and teeth	鈣	钙
calculus (n)	a stone found in the body, esp. bladder, kidneys, urethra, and ureter; gallstone; kidney stone	（結）石	（结）石
calf (n) (m)	the fleshy, muscular back part of the human leg between the knee and ankle	腓腸，小腿肚	腓肠，小腿肚
callus (n)	a localized thickening and enlargement of the skin	胼胝	胼胝
calm down (v)	to become quiet; to lack or restrict movement; to become peaceful	使平靜	使平静
calorie (n)	any of several approximately equal units of heat, each measured as the quantity of heat required to raise the temperature of 1 gram of water 1 degree Celsius	卡路里	卡路里
cancer (n)	a disease in which cells grow and reproduce without regulation, these cells have a tendency to spread to other cells of the body	癌	癌
candidiasis (n)	a specific fungus infection	念珠菌病	念珠菌病
cane (n)	a stick used as an aid in walking	扶杖	扶杖
canister (n)	a container used to hold fluid	罐	罐
capillary (n)	the end of the smallest artery and the beginning of the smallest vein; the smallest blood vessel in the body	毛細管	毛细管

English/Chinese Medical Glossary - C

capitated service (n)	services covered under a capitated health plan; see *capitation*	計酬服務	计酬服务
capitation (n)	a contractual arrangement through which a health care provider or an HMO agrees to provide specified health care services to enrollees	按人收費	按人收费
capitation rate (n)	the amount paid per enrollee, per month, for services to be provided at risk.	按人收費率	按人收费率
capsule (n)	1. a soluble container enclosing a dose of an oral medicine; 2. an envelope that encloses an organ or part in the human body	囊	囊
capsulitis (n)	inflammation of a capsule	囊炎	囊炎
car seat (n)	a device placed in an automobile, used to secure a child (under the age of six or under 45 pounds) when the automobile is in motion	〔孩童〕車輛座椅	〔孩童〕车辆座椅
carbohydrates (n)	a group of chemical compounds, including sugars and starches; major energy source of the body; also see *blood sugar*	碳水化合物	碳水化合物
carbon dioxide (n)	a colorless, odorless gas exhaled by humans as waste	二氧化碳	二氧化碳
carbon monoxide (n)	a poisonous gas found in the exhaust of a car	一氧化碳	一氧化碳
carbuncle (n)	a specific inflammation or swelling of the skin that is accompanied by excretion of pus	癰	痈
carcinogen (n)	any substance that causes or increases the risk of developing cancer	致癌物	致癌物
carcinogenic (adj)	of, or pertaining to any substance that causes or increases the risk of developing cancer	致癌的	致癌的

English/Chinese Medical Glossary - C

carcinoma (n)	a malignant new growth made up of cells tending to enter the surrounding tissues and spread throughout the body	癌	癌
cardiac (adj)	pertaining to the heart	心臟的	心脏的
cardiac arrest (n)	a sudden stop of effective pumping of the heart	心搏停止	心搏停止
cardiac catheterization (n)	a surgical procedure where a slender, flexible tube is inserted into the heart	心導管術	心导管术
cardiac scan (n)	a type of examination that studies heart function to assist in diagnosis	心臟掃描	心脏扫描
cardioangiography (n)	the process of creating an image of the heart and blood vessels around the heart by injecting an x-ray-visible liquid into the blood	心血管造影術	心血管造影术
cardiologist (n)	a person who studies diseases and functioning of the heart	心臟病學家	心脏病学家
cardiology (n)	the study of diseases and functioning of the heart	心臟病學	心脏病学
cardiopulmonary (adj)	pertaining to the heart and lungs	心肺的	心肺的
cardiopulmonary resuscitation (n)	a procedure employed after the heart stops beating in which cardiac massage, drugs, and mouth-to-mouth resuscitation are used to restore breathing	心肺復蘇術	心肺复苏术
cardiorespiratory (n)	relating to the heart and lungs and their functions	心和肺的	心和肺的
cardiovascular disease (n)	disease affecting the heart or blood vessels	心血管疾病	心血管疾病
cardiovascular system (n)	of, or pertaining to the heart and blood vessels / circulatory system	心血管系統	心血管系统
care management (n)	a coordinated system of health-care services	護理管理	护理管理
caries (n)	the molecular decay or death of a bone	骨瘍	骨疡
carotid artery (n)	one of two arteries supplying blood to the neck and head	頸動脈	颈动脉

English/Chinese Medical Glossary - C

carpal tunnel syndrome (n)	pain or loss of sensation in the hand and wrist caused by damage or overuse of the wrist	腕管綜合征	腕管综合征
carrier (n)	a person who harbors a pathogen, and may transmit disease to others, without showing signs and symptoms of infection	帶菌者	带菌者
cartilage (n)	a tough white connective tissue attached to the surfaces of bones	軟骨	软骨
case (n)	a situation, state of affairs, condition; a situation that requires examination	病例	病例
case management (n)	method of managing health care services by which the medical, psycho-social, and other services are coordinated by one entity	病例管理	病例管理
cashier (n)	the person in a business in charge of paying and receiving money	出納員	出纳员
cast (plaster) (n)	a rigid dressing, usually made of gauze and plaster of Paris, as for a broken bone	石(膏)	石(膏)
castration (n)	the removal of the testicles or ovaries	閹	阉
casualty (n)	death of an individual; fatality	傷亡	伤亡
cataract (n)	opacity in the lens of the eye, impairing vision or causing blindness	白內障	白内障
catheter (n)	a tubular, flexible, surgical instrument for withdrawing fluids (or introducing fluids into) a cavity of the body	導管	导管
catheterization (n)	the employment or passage of a catheter	導管插入術	导管插入术
catheterize (v)	to introduce a slender, flexible tube into a bodily channel, such as a vein	插入導管	插入导管
causal (adj)	pertaining to a cause; directed against a cause	原因的	原因的

English/Chinese Medical Glossary - C

caustic (adj)	capable of burning, corroding, dissolving, or otherwise eating away by chemical action	腐蝕性的	腐蚀性的
cavity (dental) (n)	a pitted area in a tooth caused by caries	蛀牙	蛀牙
cecum (n)	the first part of the large intestine	盲腸	盲肠
cell (n)	the smallest structural unit of an organism that is capable of independent functioning	細胞	细胞
cell membrane (n)	the structure enveloping a cell	細胞膜	细胞膜
Centers for Disease Control (CDC) (n)	a federal agency responsible for protecting the health and safety of people by developing and applying prevention and control of disease, injury, and disability	疾病控制中心	疾病控制中心
cereal (n) (m)	a seed or grain high in starch and carbohydrates	穀類	谷类
cerebral (adj)	of, or pertaining to the cerebrum or the brain	大腦的	大脑的
cerebral palsy (n)	impaired muscular power and coordination due to brain damage, usually occurring at or before birth	大腦性麻痹	大脑性麻痹
cerebrospinal (adj)	pertaining to the brain and spinal cord	腦脊髓的	脑脊髓的
cerebrovascular (adj)	pertaining to the blood vessels of the cerebrum, or brain	腦血管的	脑血管的
cerebrum (n)	the largest section of the brain	大腦	大脑
certificate (n)	an official document recording an event, achievement, or status	證明（書）	证明（书）
Certificate of Coverage (COC) (n)	a description of the benefits included in a carrier's plan; the certificate of coverage is required by state laws and represents the coverage provided under the contract issued to the employer; the certificate is provided to the employee	保險覆蓋範圍證書	保险覆盖范围证书

English/Chinese Medical Glossary - C

Certified Case Manager (CCM) (n)	a designation given to healthcare professionals what have formal training and "hands on" experience in the provision of case management services and processes	病例管理員 (CCM)	病例管理员 (CCM)
Certified Nurse Anesthetist (n)	a person licensed to assist an anesthesiologist	註冊麻醉護士	注册麻醉护士
Certified Nurse Midwife (n)	a person licensed to assist a pregnancy	註冊助產護士	注册助产护士
Certified Nurse's Assistant (CNA) (n)	CNA assists the RN in the patient's care	註冊護士助理 (CNA)	注册护士助理 (CNA)
cervical (adj)	pertaining to the neck, or to the neck of any organ or structure	頸的	颈的
cervical cancer (n)	cancer of the cervix, cancer of the entrance to the womb (uterus)	子宮頸癌	子宫颈癌
cervix (n)	the constricted part of an organ, especially the opening into the uterus	頸，子宮頸	颈，子宫颈
cesarean section (n)	a surgical incision through the abdominal wall and uterus, performed to extract an unborn baby	剖腹產術	剖腹产术
chamber (n)	a closed space, usually referring to a section of the heart	腔	腔
chancre (n)	a dull-red, painless ulcer that is the first evidence of syphilis	下疳	下疳
change your eating style (v)	alter or vary the way in which food is consumed	改變飲食習慣	改变饮食习惯
chart (n)	a sheet presenting information in the form of graphs or tables, esp. information about a particular patient	病例	病例
check up (n)	a visit to a doctor's office for an interview and physical examination	檢查	检查
cheek (n)	the fleshy part of either side of the face below the eye and between the nose and ear	面頰	面颊

English/Chinese Medical Glossary - C

cheekbone (n)	the bone just below the eye and above the fleshy part of the cheek	顴骨	顴骨
chemistry (n)	the scientific study of organic and inorganic elementary compounds and molecules	化學	化学
chemotherapy (n)	the treatment of disease, esp. cancer, by means of chemicals	化學療法	化学疗法
chest (n)	the part of the body between the neck and the abdomen, enclosed by the ribs and the breastbone	胸腔	胸腔
chest hair (n)	hair located on the chest	胸毛	胸毛
chest pain (n)	an unpleasant sensation in the chest	胸痛	胸痛
chest x-ray (n)	a photograph of the chest, using x-rays, which produces an image of the lungs, ribs, and other aspects of the thorax	胸部 x 光照片	胸部 x 光照片
chew (v)	to bite and mash food with the teeth	咀嚼	咀嚼
chicken pox (n)	a very contagious disease, usually of young children, characterized by skin eruption and slight fever	水痘	水痘
Chief Medical Director (n)	a physician responsible for policy and procedures, and approval and denial of health-care services provided by a health plan or health network; He/She is also responsible for administrative matters of the health plan or health network related to health-care service delivery (in some health plans or health networks he/she may be called Medical Director)	首席醫療顧問	首席医疗顾问
child abuse (n)	the illegal act of physically or mentally injuring a child	虐待兒童	虐待儿童

English/Chinese Medical Glossary - C

Child Health and Disability Prevention (CHDP) (n)	a program which covers screening and diagnostic services to determine physical and mental defects in children under the age of 21 and to ascertain health care treatment and other measures to correct or ameliorate any defects and chronic conditions discovered	兒童健康與殘疾預防 (CHDP)	儿童健康与残疾预防（CHDP）
childbirth (n)	the process of giving birth, or passing a child through the birth canal	分娩	分娩
chills (n)	a sensation of coldness, as with a fever	受寒	受寒
chin (n)	the central forward portion of the lower jaw	頦	颏
chiropractic (n)	a system of therapy in which disease is considered the result of incorrect alignment of bones causing poor function of the nerves; adjustments of the backbone and other structures is the preferred method of treatment	按摩療法	按摩疗法
chiropractor (n)	a person who applies chiropractic therapy	按摩技士	按摩技士
choke (v)	to prevent normal breathing, esp. by blocking the windpipe or by polluting the air	氣阻	气阻
cholecystectomy (n)	surgical removal of the gallbladder	膽囊切除術	胆囊切除术
cholera (n)	an acute, often fatal disease causing diarrhea, vomiting, cramps, and collapse	霍亂	霍乱
cholesterol (n)	a pearly, fat-like substance that is a major cause of heart disease	膽固醇	胆固醇
chronic (adj)	persisting over a long period of time	慢性的	慢性的
chronic bronchitis (n)	a continuous inflammation of the bronchi	慢性支氣管炎	慢性支气管炎

English/Chinese Medical Glossary - C

chronic obstructive pulmonary disease (n)	a process that decreases the functioning of the lungs caused by numerous diseases	慢性阻塞性肺病	慢性阻塞性肺病
circulation (n)	the movement of blood through bodily vessels as a result of the heart's pumping action	循環	循环
circulatory system (n)	the vessels, arteries, and veins, through which blood moves	循環系統	循环系统
circumcision (n)	the act of removing a section of the male or female external sexual organs	包皮環切術	包皮环切术
cirrhosis (n)	a chronic disease of the liver marked by destruction and loss of liver cells leading to liver failure	〔肝〕硬變	（肝）硬变
classic (adj)	first class of rank; standard; well-known and typical	典型的	典型的
classification (n)	the act or result of arranging or organizing according to class or category	分類	分类
clavicle (n)	a bone that links the shoulder to the chest	鎖骨	锁骨
clearance (n) (m)	the process of clearing; the rate at which a substance is removed from the blood	清除	清除
client (n)	a person served by or utilizing the services of a social agency	客戶	客戶
clinic (n)	an institution associated with a hospital or medical school that deals chiefly with outpatients; a medical establishment run by several specialists working in cooperation	門診處，診所	门诊，诊所
clitoral (adj)	pertaining to the clitoris	陰蒂的	阴蒂的
clitoris (n)	a small, erectile female sexual organ similar to the penis	陰蒂	阴蒂
clogged artery (n)	an obstructed or blocked artery	動脈阻塞	动脉阻塞
clot (blood) (v)	to form into clots	凝結(血)	凝结（血）
clot (n)	a thick mass or lump usually found in blood vessels	凝塊	凝块

English/Chinese Medical Glossary - C

cloudy urine (n)	urine that is not clear	渾濁尿	浑浊尿
clubbed fingers (n)	a condition where soft tissue in the fingers increases and fingernails curve in an abnormal way	杵狀指	杵状指
coagulation (n)	the process of clot formation	凝結	凝结
coccyx (n)	a small bone at the base of the spinal column	尾骨	尾骨
cold (illness) (n) (m)	common cold, a viral respiratory infection characterized by fever, chills, coughing, and sneezing	受寒 (感冒)	受寒（感冒）
cold sore (n)	a small ulcer or blister on the lips, usually accompanying a cold or fever	感冒瘡	感冒疮
cold sweat (n)	sweat and chills happening at the same time, usually caused by fear, pain, or shock	冷汗	冷汗
cold turkey (n)	a slang phrase used when people quit using an addictive substance all at once, without a period of gradual adjustment	突然停止	突然停止
colic (n)	acute pain in the abdomen, caused by spasm, obstruction, or widening of the intestine	絞痛	绞痛
colitis (n)	inflammation of the colon	結腸炎	结肠炎
collapse (v)	to fall down; to cease to function; break down suddenly in strength or health	虛脫	虚脱
collar bone (n)	the clavicle	鎖骨	锁骨
colon (n)	the large intestine extending from the cecum to the rectum	結腸	结肠
colonoscopy (n)	a procedure using a slender tubular instrument with a small light on the end for inspection of the colon	結腸鏡檢查	结肠镜检查
color blindness (n)	an inability to see one or more colors	色盲	色盲
colorectal cancer (n)	cancer of the colon and rectum	結腸直腸癌	结肠直肠癌
colposcopy (n)	the examination of the vaginal and cervical tissues	陰道窺鏡檢查	阴道窥镜检查

English/Chinese Medical Glossary - C

coma (n)	a deep, prolonged unconsciousness, usually the result of injury, disease, or poison	昏迷	昏迷
comatose (n)	pertaining to or affected with a coma	昏迷狀態	昏迷状态
combination (n)	a result or product of combining	結合	结合
comfort (v)	to relieve or soothe pain during a difficult period	安慰	安慰
communicable disease (n)	a disease that is capable of being passed between people	傳染性疾病	传染性疾病
communication device (n)	a tool to help a person talk to another person	通訊設備	通讯设备
communication services (n)	services provided to help a person talk to another person	通訊服務	通讯服务
Community Alcohol & Drug Prevention (n)	public programs that offer education, support, and outreach resources to increase awareness of the dangers of alcohol and drug abuse	社區酒精和毒品預防	社区酒精和毒品预防
Community Clinic (n)	a place in the neighborhood where people can come for routine health care services	社區診所	社区诊所
compatible (n)	capable of living or performing in pleasant combination with another or others; capable of forming a stable system	相容	相容
compensation (n)	the act of making up for or offsetting; counterbalance	補償	补偿
complain (v)	to express disappointment or dissatisfaction	抱怨	抱怨
complaint (n)	an expression of disappointment or dissatisfaction	抱怨	抱怨
complementary (n)	forming or serving as a complement; completing	補充	补充
complex (adj)	complicated, not simple	複雜的	复杂的
complication (n)	a condition occurring during another disease and aggravating it	併發症	并发症
component (n)	a constituent element or part, as of a system	成分；組元	成分；组元

English/Chinese Medical Glossary - C

compress (n) (m)	a soft pad of gauze or other material applied to a part of the body to control bleeding or, moistened with water or medication, to reduce pain or infection	敷布	敷布
computer axial tomography (n)	a diagnostic image of internal organs and soft tissue; also CAT scan	電腦掃描	电脑扫描
conceive (v) (m)	to become pregnant	受孕	受孕
concentration (n) (m)	increase in strength by evaporation; the act of bringing a set of things closely together	濃縮	浓缩
conception (n) (m)	the first steps or beginning of pregnancy	受孕	受孕
concomitant (n)	accompanying; accessory; joined with another	附隨物	附随物
concrete (n) (m)	solid, tangible	凝結體	凝结体
concurrent review (n)	an assessment that determines medical necessity or appropriateness of services as they are rendered, such as an assessment of the need for continued inpatient care for hospitalized patients	住院期間審核	住院期间审核
concussion (n)	a severe injury or shock, esp. to the brain	（腦）震盪	（脑）震荡
condition (n) (m)	1. the state of being or health of a person; 2. a specific ailment or disease	情況	情况
condom (n)	a sheath, usually made of thin rubber, designed to cover the penis during sexual intercourse to prevent pregnancy or the exchange of diseases	避孕套	避孕套
conduction (n)	the transfer of sound waves, heat, nervous impulses, or electricity	傳導	传导
confidential (adj)	done or communicated in secret	機密的	机密的

English/Chinese Medical Glossary - C

confusion (n)	disturbed orientation in regard to time, place, or person	精神錯亂	精神错乱
congenital (adj)	of, or pertaining to a medical condition existing at, and usually before birth	先天的	先天的
congenital heart disease (n)	a heart disease that existed at birth but is not hereditary	先天性心臟病	先天性心脏病
congested, stuffed up (adj) (m)	having an accumulation of fluid in the lungs or nose	堵塞	堵塞
congestion (n) (m)	excessive or abnormal accumulation of fluid in a part	充血	充血
congestive heart failure (n)	an enlarging and weakening of the heart caused by various heart diseases	心力衰竭	心力衰竭
conjunctivitis (n)	inflammation of the mucous membrane that lines the inner surface of the eyelid and the exposed surface of the eyeball; pink eye	結膜炎	结膜炎
conscious (n)	having an awareness of one's own existence, sensations, and thoughts, and of one's environment; capable of thought	意識	意识
consent (n)	to agree; to be of the same mind or opinion	同意	同意
conservative (adj)	cautious	保守的	保守的
conserve (v)	to keep in a safe or sound state, preserve from change or destruction	保存	保存
Consolidated Omnibus Budget Reconciliation Act (COBRA) (n)	A federal law that, among other things, requires employers to offer continued health insurance coverage to certain employees and their beneficiaries whose group health insurance coverage has been terminated	統一綜合財務調節法案（COBRA）	统一综合财务调节法案（COBRA）
constipated (adj)	experiencing difficult, incomplete, or infrequent release of feces	患便秘症的	患便秘症的
constitutional (adj) (m)	affecting the whole body; not local	全身的	全身的

English/Chinese Medical Glossary - C

consulting nurse (n)	a nurse that provides medical advice	諮詢護士	咨询护士
contact (n)	the coming together or touching of two objects or surfaces; a mutual touching of two bodies or persons	接觸	接触
contact lens (n)	a thin corrective lens that fits on the eyeball	隱形眼鏡	隐形眼镜
contagious (adj)	passing by direct or indirect contact; carrying or capable of carrying disease	接觸傳染的	接触传染的
contamination (n)	the act of polluting, soiling, or making something dirty; the act of giving something the ability to transfer a disease or cause an infection	污染	污染
contraception (n)	the prevention of conception or pregnancy	避孕	避孕
contraceptive (n)	an agent that diminishes the likelihood of or prevents one from becoming pregnant	避孕的	避孕的
contract (a disease) (v)	to acquire a disease	得病	得病
contracting providers (n)	a physician, nurse, technician, teacher, researcher, hospital, home health agency, nursing home, or any other individual or institution that an entity contracts with for medical services	締約提供者	缔约提供者
contraction (n)	a shortening or reduction in size, esp. the shortening of muscle	收縮	收缩
contracture (n)	a drawing together, as of muscle or scar tissue, resulting in distortion or deformity	攣縮	挛缩
contraindication (n)	any condition, especially any condition of disease, which renders some particular line of treatment improper or undesirable	禁忌症	禁忌症
contrast medium (n)	a substance that is introduced into or around a structure which allows a structure to become visible through x-ray	造影劑	造影剂

English/Chinese Medical Glossary - C

English	Definition	Traditional	Simplified
control (v)	1. to exercise restraint; 2. to have direct influence over; 3. to regulate, limit	節制，限制	节制，限制
controlled drugs (n)	depressant and stimulant drugs that are frequently abused and must be prescribed for use by a physician	受管制藥品	受管制药品
contusion (n)	a bruise, an injury of a part without a break in the skin	挫傷	挫伤
convalescence (n)	the stage of recovery following an attack of disease, a surgical operation, or an injury	恢復期	恢复期
conventional (adj)	traditional or customary	常規的	常规的
conversion (n) (m)	the development of repressed ideas or impulses in motor or sensory disorders such as paralysis	轉化	转化
convulsion (n)	a violent involuntary contraction or a series of rapid movements	抽搐	抽搐
cool-down (n)	a gradual decrease in activity at the end of an exercise session where the heart rate lowers to resting levels (60-80 beats per minute); muscle stretching and limbering exercises typically are performed to reduce the risk of developing delayed muscle soreness	降溫	降温
coordinates a person's health care (v)	to link one service to another in order to take care of a person's health	協調病人的健康護理	协调病人的健康护理
coordination (n)	the harmonious functioning of interrelated organs and parts	協調	协调

English/Chinese Medical Glossary - C

coordination of benefits (COB) (v)	a provision in a contract that applies when a person is covered under more than one group medical program. It requires that payment of benefits will be coordinated by all programs to eliminate over-insurance or duplication of benefits	協調福利	协调福利
coordination of clinical care (v)	the mechanisms ensuring that the patient and clinicians have access to, and take into consideration, all required information regarding the patient's conditions and treatments to ensure that the patient receives appropriate health-care services	協調臨床護理	协调临床护理
cope (v)	to face and deal with something that is difficult or challenging	應對	应对
copyright (n)	the exclusive legal right to reproduce, publish, and sell the matter and form (as of a literary, musical, or artistic work)	版權	版权
cornea (n)	the transparent structure forming the anterior or front part of the eye; a uniformly thick, nearly circular structure covering the lens of the eye	角膜	角膜
coronary (adj)	of, or pertaining to the heart, esp. the blood vessels, nerves, and ligaments in and around the heart	冠狀的	冠状的
coronary artery (n)	one of the two arteries that supply blood to the heart	冠狀動脈	冠状动脉
coronary artery disease (n)	a pathology of the arteries that supply blood to the heart	冠狀動脈疾病	冠状动脉疾病
coronary bypass surgery (n)	a surgical procedure that provides a new passage for a blocked coronary artery	冠狀動脈搭橋手術	冠状动脉搭橋手术

English/Chinese Medical Glossary - C

coronary care unit (n)	a specially equipped area of a hospital providing intensive nursing and medical care for patients who have acute heart disease	冠心病護理病房	冠心病护理病房
correction (n)	the act or process of removing errors or mistakes	矯正	矫正
correlation (n)	a causal, complementary, parallel, or reciprocal relationship, esp. a structural, functional, or qualitative correspondence between two comparable items	相關	相关
correspond (n)	to be in agreement, harmony, or conformity; to be consistent or compatible	符合	符合
corticosteroid (n)	any of the steroids made in the adrenal cortex	皮質類固醇	皮质类固醇
cosmetic (adj) (m)	serving to beautify the body; decorative rather than functional	美容的	美容的
cosmetic (n) (m)	a preparation, such as skin cream, designed to beautify the body by direct application	美容劑	美容剂
cosmetic surgery (n)	a surgical procedure that corrects physical defects or non-functional aspects of the human anatomy	整容手術	整容手术
cotton (n)	thread or cloth manufactured from cotton fiber	棉花	棉花
cotton balls (n)	a small weave of cotton used to clean the skin	棉球	棉球
cough (v)	to expel air from the lungs suddenly and noisily	咳嗽	咳嗽
cough drops (n)	a small, often medicated and sweetened lozenge or candy taken to ease coughing or soothe a sore throat	喉糖	喉糖
cough syrup (n)	a medicated and sweetened liquid taken to ease coughing or soothe a sore throat	止咳糖漿	止咳糖浆
counselor (n)	a person who gives counsel; adviser	顧問	顾问

English/Chinese Medical Glossary - C

English	Definition	Traditional	Simplified
coverage (insurance) (n)	the extent of protection afforded by an insurance policy	（保險）範圍	（保险）范围
covered services (n)	health care services which are reasonable and necessary to protect life, to prevent significant illness or significant disability, or alleviate severe pain through the diagnosis or treatment of disease, illness, or injury, subject to utilization controls	承保服務	承保服务
CPT codes/coding system (n)	universally accepted billing codes [CPT = Current Procedural Terminology] utilized by healthcare providers for healthcare services and durable medical equipment (DME)	現時程式技術編號/編碼系統	现时程序技术编号/编码系统
cramp (n)	a sudden involuntary muscular contraction causing severe pain, often occurring in the leg or shoulder as the result of strain or chill	痛性痙攣	痛性痉挛
cranium (n)	the portion of the skull enclosing the brain	顱	颅
crawl (v)	to move by using the hands and knees	爬行	爬行
credentialing (n)	a process of review to approve a provider who applies to participate in a health plan; specific criteria and prerequisites are applied in determining initial and ongoing participation in the health plan	證照審核	证照审核
crippled (adj)	partly disabled or lame	殘疾的	残疾的
crisis (n) (m)	a sudden paroxysmal intensification of symptoms in the course of a disease	危象	危象

English/Chinese Medical Glossary - C

criteria (n)	systematically developed, objective, and quantifiable statements used to assess the appropriateness of specific health care decisions, services, and outcomes	標準	标准
criterion (n)	a standard by which something may be judged	判斷標準	判断标准
critical condition (n)	of, or pertaining, to a crisis	臨界狀態	临界状态
Crohn's Disease (n)	a chronic intestinal disease associated with inflammation of the small intestines	克羅恩氏病，局部性迴腸炎	克罗恩氏病，局部性迴肠炎
cross-eyed (adj)	having eyes that look in toward the nose	斜視的	斜视的
crotch (n)	the region of the angle formed by the junction of the legs	胯部	胯部
croup (n)	a pathological condition affecting the larynx in children, characterized by respiratory difficulty and a harsh cough	哮吼	哮吼
crown (dental) (n) (m)	an artificial substitute for the part of the tooth above the gum line	（牙）冠	（牙）冠
crutch (n)	a device used to aid a paralyzed, weak, or injured person, usually a long stick or staff placed under the arm for support	拐杖	拐杖
cryosurgery (n)	the selective exposure of tissues to extreme cold to bring about cell destruction	冷凍手術	冷冻手术
cryotherapy (n)	application of liquid nitrogen; the use of low temperatures in medical therapy	冷療法	冷疗法
crystallization (n)	the formation of crystals	結晶	结晶
crystals (n)	a three-dimensional atomic, ionic, or molecular structure consisting of periodically repeated, identically constituted, congruent unit cells	晶體	晶体
culture (n) (m)	the growing of microorganisms in a small dish	培養	培养

English/Chinese Medical Glossary - C

cumulative (adj)	increasing or growing by accumulation or successive additions	蓄積的	蓄积的
curative (n)	an agent that helps overcome a disease and promote recovery	治療物	治疗物
cure (n)	a method or course of medical treatment used to restore health; an agent, such as a drug, that restores health; remedy	治療	治疗
curettage (n)	the removal of growths or other material from the wall of a cavity or other surface	刮除術	刮除术
curve (n)	a line that deviates from straightness in a smooth, continuous fashion	曲線	曲线
Customer Service Department (n)	a group of people organized and working together under a leader, and responsible for providing services (information, referral, and problem resolution) to patients, doctors, community, advocates, and others as needed	客戶服務部	客户服务部
cut (n)	the result of cutting; an incision; the act of incising, severing, or separating	切割	切割
cut (v)	to penetrate with a sharp edge; strike a narrow opening in	切割	切割
cutaneous (adj)	pertaining to the skin; dermal; dermic	皮的	皮的
cuticle (n)	the strip of hardened skin at the base of a fingernail or toenail	表皮	表皮
cyanosis (n)	a bluish discoloration of the skin, resulting from inadequate oxygenation of the blood	發紫紺	发紫紺
cycle (n)	a time interval in which a characteristic, esp. a regularly repeated, event or sequence of events occurs	週期	周期

English/Chinese Medical Glossary - C

cyclic (adj)	of, or pertaining to, or occurring in a cycle or cycles	週期的	周期的
cycloplegia (n)	inability to focus because of paralysis of the ciliary muscles of the eye	睫狀肌麻痹	睫状肌麻痹
cyst (n)	any closed cavity or sac	囊	囊
cystic fibrosis (n)	a congenital disease causing chronic obstructive pulmonary disease and problems with the pancreas	囊性纖維病	囊性纤维病
cystitis (n)	inflammation of the urinary bladder	膀胱炎	膀胱炎
cystoscopy (n)	direct visual examination of the urinary tract with a tubular instrument fitted with a light	膀胱鏡檢查	膀胱镜检查

Notes

English/Chinese Medical Glossary - D

damage (n)	impairment of the usefulness or value of person or property; harm	損傷	损伤
dandruff (n)	white scaly skin that develops on and is shed from the head	頭皮屑	头皮屑
danger (n)	a situation or condition that is harmful and may cause injury	危險	危险
dangerous (adj)	of, or pertaining to a situation or condition that is harmful and may cause injury	危險的	危险的
dazed (adj)	in a confused mental state	茫然的	茫然的
deaf (adj)	partially or completely incapable of hearing	聾的	聋的
deafness (n)	the state of being partially or completely incapable of hearing	聾	聋
death (n)	the act of dying; state of being dead	死亡	死亡
death certificate (n)	an official document recording the time, date, and location of a person's death	死亡證明	死亡证明
decay (v)	to decompose, rot	腐爛	腐烂
decompensation (n)	any process or mechanism to adjust or compensate; process of getting worse	代償失調	代偿失调
decompression (n)	the act or process of relieving pressure; a surgical procedure used to relieve pressure on an organ or part	減壓	减压
decongestant (n)	a medication or treatment that breaks up congestion, as of the sinuses	減充血劑 減輕鼻塞劑	减充血剂 减轻鼻塞剂
deep (adj)	extending far downward below a surface; extending far inward from an outer surface	深的	深的
deep breathing (v)	the act or process of slowly allowing air to come through the nostrils and fill up the lower abdomen and then having the air escape through pursed lips	深呼吸	深呼吸
defecate (v)	to excrete or release feces from the bowels	排便	排便

English/Chinese Medical Glossary - D

deferred (v)	to delay an action or proceeding	延遲	延迟
defibrillation (n)	the act of correcting an irregular heart beat by applying electric shock across the chest	除顫	除颤
deficiency (n)	a lack of an essential quality or element	缺乏	缺乏
deficit (n)	the amount by which something, as a sum of money, falls short of the required or expected amount; shortage	短缺	短缺
deformity (n)	the state of being misshapen or disfigured	畸形	畸形
degeneration (n)	the process of losing function, or a decline from an original state	退化	退化
degenerative (n)	undergoing a decline, as in function or nature, from a former or original state	退行性	退行性
degenerative disc (n)	a condition characterized by a decline in the function of the discs in joints, esp. in the spine	椎間盤退變性疾病	椎间盘退变性疾病
degenerative joint disease (n)	a condition characterized by a decline in function of the joints, osteoarthritis	關節變性疾病	关节变性疾病
degradation (n)	the act or process of decomposing or lowering by wear	分解	分解
dehydrate (v)	to remove water from the body	脫水	脱水
dehydration (n)	the condition that results from excessive loss of body water	脫水	脱水
delirium (n)	an acute, reversible organic mental disorder characterized by reduced ability to maintain attention	妄想	妄想
deliver, give birth (v)	to assist in giving birth; to assist or aid in the birth of	接生，助產	接生，助产
delivery room (n)	the location where a woman gives birth	產房	产房
delivery, childbirth (n)	the act of giving birth	分娩	分娩
delusion (n)	a false opinion or idea	妄想	妄想

English/Chinese Medical Glossary - D

dementia (n)	a mental disorder characterized by a general loss of intellectual abilities	癡呆	痴呆
dental floss (n)	a strong waxed or unwaxed thread used to clean areas between the teeth	牙線	牙线
dental hygiene (n)	a term used for maintaining teeth and the oral cavity by brushing, flossing, and visiting a dentist regularly	口腔衛生	口腔卫生
dental plaque (n)	a soft, thin film of food debris and other substances deposited on the teeth	牙垢	牙垢
dentist (n)	a person whose profession is dentistry	牙醫	牙医
dentistry (n)	the diagnosis, prevention, and treatment of diseases of the teeth and related structures	牙科〔學〕	牙科（学）
denture (n)	a set of artificial teeth	假牙	托牙，假牙
dependent (n)	contingent upon something or someone else	依靠	依靠
depersonalization (n)	alteration in the perception of the self so that the usual sense of one's own reality is lost	人格解體	人格解体
depigmentation (n)	removal or loss of pigment	褪色	褪色
depletion (n)	the act or process of emptying; removal of fluid, such as blood	排除	排除
depolarization (n)	the process or act of neutralizing polarity	去極化	去极化
depress (v)	definition?	壓下，使抑鬱	压下，使抑郁
depression (n)	a condition of lowered spirits or sadness	抑鬱	抑郁
deprivation (n)	loss or absence of parts, organs, powers, or things that are needed	喪失	丧失
dermatitis (n)	inflammation of the skin	皮膚炎	皮肤炎
dermatologist (n)	a person whose profession is dermatology	皮膚科醫生	皮肤科医生
dermatology (n)	the medical study of the physiology and pathology of the skin	皮膚病學	皮肤病学

English/Chinese Medical Glossary - D

dermatosis (n)	any skin disease, especially one not characterized by inflammation	皮膚病	皮肤病
descending colon (n)	the third section of the large intestine that moves feces and waste downward towards the rectum	降結腸	降结肠
desensitization (n)	the act of rendering less sensitive or insensitive, as to light or pain; reduction of allergic reaction	脫敏	脱敏
dessert (n)	any of various foods that are often high in fat and sugar, usually eaten after a meal	甜點	甜点
detection (n)	the act of finding something or a substance through experiments or observation	檢測	检测
detergent (n)	a cleansing substance made from chemical compounds rather than from fats and lye	去污劑	去污剂
detoxification (n)	the act or process of counteracting or destroying the toxic properties of a substance	解毒作用	解毒作用
dextrose (n)	sugars found in animal and plant tissue and derived from starch; also see *carbohydrate*	葡萄糖	葡萄糖
diabetes (n)	a general term referring to disorders characterized by excessive urine discharge and persistent thirst; most commonly, it refers to a condition associated with high blood sugar	糖尿病	糖尿病
diabetes management (n)	the control of blood sugar (blood glucose) levels by regular exercise, eating a healthy diet and taking medications as prescribed, if needed	糖尿病管理	糖尿病管理
diabetic (adj)	of, relating to, or having diabetes	糖尿病的	糖尿病的

English/Chinese Medical Glossary - D

diabetic retinopathy (n)	a common complication of diabetes affecting the blood vessels in the retina (the thin membrane that covers the back of the eye); if untreated, it may lead to blindness; if diagnosed and treated promptly, blindness is usually preventable	糖尿病視網膜病	糖尿病视网膜病
diagnosis (n)	the act or process of identifying or determining the nature of a disease through examination; also the result of this process	診斷	诊断
diagnosis related groups (DRGs) (n)	a system of classification for inpatient hospital services based on principal diagnosis, secondary diagnosis, surgical procedures, age, sex, and presence of complications; this system of classification is used as a financing mechanism to reimburse hospital and other providers for services rendered	診斷關聯群 (DRG)	诊断关联群 (DRG)
diagnostic test (n)	any of various tests used to detect a disease or determine a patient's medical condition	診斷檢查	诊断检查
dialysis (n)	the separation of smaller molecules from larger molecules; this technique is commonly used to remove waste or toxins from the body in patients whose kidneys do not work well	透析	透析
diameter (n)	length of a straight line passing through the center of a circle and connecting opposite points on its circumference	直徑	直径
diaper (n)	a folded piece of cloth or other absorbent material placed between a baby's legs and pinned at the waist	尿布	尿布

English/Chinese Medical Glossary - D

diaper rash (n)	a skin irritation or redness caused by excessive use of a diaper	尿布疹	尿布疹
diaphragm (n)	a contraceptive used in family planning that blocks the opening to the uterus	子宮帽	子宫帽
diaphragm (n)	a muscular wall separating abdominal and thoracic cavities, which helps in breathing	橫膈膜	横膈膜
diarrhea (n)	a condition of having feces that contains abnormally high levels of water	腹瀉	腹泻
diastole (n)	the period when the heart is relaxed and is filling with blood	舒張	舒张
diastolic (adj)	of, or pertaining to the diastole	舒張的	舒张的
die (v)	to cease living; to expire	死	死
diet (n)	the usual food and drink of a person; a regulated selection of foods, esp. as prescribed for medical reasons	日常飲食	日常饮食
dietitian (n)	a person specializing in the study of diet and dieting as it relates to health and hygiene	飲食學家	饮食学家
difficulty (n)	the condition or quality of being hard to do, achieve, or perform	困難	困难
diffusion (n)	the process of becoming widely spread	擴散	扩散
digestion (n)	the primary bodily process by which food is decomposed into simple, absorbable substances used in proper body function	消化	消化
digestive (adj)	pertaining to digestion	消化的	消化的
digestive system (n)	the system of organs in the body involved in digestion, including the large intestines, small intestines, and accessory glands, including salivary glands, liver, and pancreas	消化系統	消化系统

English/Chinese Medical Glossary - D

dilation (n)	the condition in which an opening is enlarged or stretched beyond the normal dimensions; the act or process of enlarging or stretching	擴張	扩张
dilation and curettage (n)	a surgical procedure that expands the cervical canal of the uterus so that the surface lining of the uterus can be scraped	擴張及刮除術	扩张及刮除术
diminished (adj)	a condition of having been reduced or made smaller	減少了的	减少了的
diphtheria (n)	an acute contagious disease caused by infection and characterized by difficulty in breathing, high fever, and weakness	白喉	白喉
disability (n)	a disabled condition; incapacity; something that disables; handicap	勞動能力喪失	劳动能力丧失
disable (v) (m)	to weaken or destroy the normal physical or mental abilities of; to incapacitate	使殘疾	使残疾
discharge (n)	something that is discharged, released, or emitted	排出物	排出物
discharge (v)	to relieve of a burden or of contents; to release, such as to discharge pus; to release from confinement, such as to discharge from a hospital	排出；出院	排出；出院
discharge planning (v)	the comprehensive evaluation of a patient's health needs in order to arrange for appropriate care after discharge from an institutional clinical care setting	出院計劃	出院计划
discomfort (n)	an unpleasant or painful sensation; a condition of not feeling good associated with a specific situation	不舒適	不舒适
disease (n)	illness or sickness often characterized by typical patient problems (symptoms) and physical findings (signs)	疾病	疾病

English/Chinese Medical Glossary - D

disinfect (v)	to clean by removing all substances that may cause an infection	消毒	消毒
disinfectant (n)	an agent that removes harmful microorganisms; applied particularly to destroy harmful microorganisms on inanimate objects	消毒劑	消毒剂
disk (n)	a thin, flat, circular plate	盤	盘
dislocate (v)	to displace a limb or organ from the normal position, esp. to displace a bone from the socket or joint	使脫臼	使脱臼
dislocated (adj)	pertaining to something that is displaced	脫臼的	脱臼的
dislocation (n)	the displacement of any part, esp. of a bone	脫位	脱位
disorientation (n)	the loss of proper bearings, or a state of mental confusion as to time, place, or identity	定向力缺失	定向力缺失
disoriented (adj)	not knowing one's position or location; confused	分不清方向的，困惑的	分不清方向的，困惑的
disseminate (v)	to scatter or distribute over a considerable area	散播	散播
dissociation (n)	the act of separating or state of being separated	分離	分离
dissolve (v)	to cause to disappear in a liquid; to break into parts	溶解	溶解
distend (v)	to swell out or expand from or as if from internal pressure	膨脹	膨胀
distention (n)	the state of being distended or enlarged; the act of distending	膨脹	膨胀
distortion (n)	the state of being twisted or bent out of a natural or normal shape or position	變形	变形
distribution (n)	specific location or arrangement of objects, or of continuing or successive events in space or time	分佈	分布

English/Chinese Medical Glossary - D

disturbance (n)	the act of breaking up or destroying the settled state of; a departure or divergence from that which is considered normal	失調	失调
diuretic (adj)	tending to increase the discharge of urine	利尿的	利尿的
diuretic (n)	a drug or agent that increases the discharge of urine	利尿劑	利尿剂
diurnal (adj)	occurring during the day	晝間的，白天的	昼间的，白天的
diverticulitis (n)	inflammation of a diverticulum, especially inflammation of the small pockets in the wall of the colon which fill with fecal material	憩室炎	憩室炎
diverticulum (n)	a pouch or sac branching out from a hollow organ or structure, such as the intestine	憩室	憩室
dizziness (n)	the sensation or feeling of whirling or tendency to fall	頭暈	头晕
dizzy (adj)	having a whirling sensation or feeling a tendency to fall	頭暈的	头晕的
doctor (n)	person trained in the healing arts and licensed to practice, esp. a physician, surgeon, dentist, or veterinarian	醫生	医生
doctor's office (n)	the location where a doctor works and meets patients	醫生辦公室	医生办公室
document (n)	an original or official paper relied upon as the basis, proof or support of something	文件	文件
domestic violence (n)	the emotional or physical force used with the intention of hurting someone typically a family member, a spouse, boyfriend or girlfriend	家庭暴力	家庭暴力

English/Chinese Medical Glossary - D

dominance (n)	the act of gaining or displaying control over someone or something else; esp. in genetics, a human trait or characteristic that is visible (as opposed to an invisible recessive trait)	優勢	优势
donor (n)	an individual person that supplies living tissue to be used in another body, such as a person who furnishes a blood transfusion	捐贈人	捐赠人
dosage (n)	determination and regulation of the size, frequency, and number of doses	劑量	剂量
dosage schedule (n)	a scheme set up to determine and regulate size, frequency, and number of doses	劑量日程表	剂量日程表
dose (n)	quantity to be administered at one time, such as a specified amount of medication	量	量
double vision (n)	seeing two images of an object when only one is present	複視	复视
double-blind (adj)	pertaining to a clinical trial or other experiment in which neither the subject nor the person administering treatment knows which treatment any particular subject is receiving	雙盲試驗	双盲试验
douche (v)	to clean or apply a medication by directing a stream or current of water against a part, esp. the vagina	灌洗	灌洗
Down's Syndrome (n)	a congenital disorder characterized by moderate to severe mental retardation, a short flattened skull, and slanting eyes	唐氏綜合症	唐氏综合症
drain (v)	to remove or empty liquid, esp. to remove fluid from a wound or internal cavity	引流	引流

English/Chinese Medical Glossary - D

drainage (n)	the withdrawal of fluids and discharges from a wound, sore or cavity	引流法	引流法
dressing (n)	the therapeutic materials applied to a wound	包紮用品	包扎用品
drop (n) (m)	a minute quantity of a substance	微量	微量
drop (v) (m)	to let something fall down	滴下	滴下
drown (v)	to kill by submerging and suffocating in water or another liquid	溺死	溺死
drowsy (adj)	dull with sleepiness; sluggish	嗜睡的	嗜睡的
drug addict (n)	a person addicted to a substance or drug	藥癮者	药瘾者
drug addiction (n)	the state of being addicted to a substance or drug	藥癮	药瘾
drug formulary (n)	a listing of prescription medications that are preferred for use by a health plan and which will be dispensed through participating pharmacies to covered persons; this list is subject to periodic review and modification	處方集	处方集
drug overdose (n)	an excessive dose, usually having harmful effects	服藥過量	服药过量
drugstore (n)	a store where prescriptions are filled and drugs and other articles are sold	藥房	药房
drunk (adj)	intoxicated with alcohol to the point of impairment of physical and mental faculties	醉的	醉的
dry heat (n)	a condition where the temperature is high but the humidity of the air is low; little water vapor in the air	乾熱	干热
dry mouth (n)	the lack of moisture or saliva in the mouth	口乾燥	口干燥
dry nose (n)	the lack of moisture or mucus in the nose	乾燥鼻	干燥鼻

English/Chinese Medical Glossary - D

English	Definition	Traditional	Simplified
duct (n)	a passage with well-defined walls, especially a tube for the passage of excretions or secretions	導管	导管
duodenal ulcer (n)	an inflammatory lesion on the first section of the small intestine	十二指腸潰瘍	十二指肠溃疡
duodenum (n)	first or proximal portion of the small intestine, extending from the pylorus to the jejunum	十二指腸	十二指肠
dura mater (n)	outermost, toughest section of membrane covering the brain and spinal cord	硬腦膜	硬脑膜
Durable Medical Equipment (DME) (n)	equipment, which can stand repeated use, that is primarily and customarily used to serve a medical purpose, generally is not useful to a person in the absence of illness or injury, and is appropriate for use at home; examples of durable medical equipment include hospital beds, wheelchairs, and oxygen equipment	耐用性醫療設備 (DME)	耐用性医疗设备（DME）
duration (n)	continuance or persistence in time; period of time during which something exists or persists	持續時間	持续时间
dust mite (n)	a very small insect that lives in house dust and commonly causes an allergic reaction	塵蟎	尘螨
dysentery (n)	any of various disorders marked by inflammation of the intestines, especially of the colon, and attended by pain in the abdomen, and stools containing blood and mucus	痢疾	痢疾
dysfunction (n)	disturbance, impairment, or abnormality of the functioning of an organ	機能障礙	机能障碍
dyslexia (n)	impairment of the ability to read	誦讀困難	诵读困难

English/Chinese Medical Glossary - D

dyspepsia (n)	disturbed digestion; indigestion	消化不良	消化不良
dysphasia (n)	impairment of speech due to brain injury	言語困難	言语困难
dystrophy (n)	any disorder arising from defective or faulty nutrition, esp. muscular dystrophy	发展不良	發展不良

Notes

English/Chinese Medical Glossary - E

ear (n)	an organ of hearing, responsible, in general, for maintaining balance as well as sensing sound, and divided in humans into the external ear, the middle ear, and the internal ear	耳	耳
ear bone (n)	one of three bones (the malleus, incus, or stapes) in the ear that assist in hearing	聽小骨	听小骨
ear canal (n)	the section of the ear leading to the middle ear	耳道	耳道
ear drops (n)	medicine administered directly into the ear, usually for healing an earache or to dissolve wax	滴耳劑	滴耳剂
ear drum (n)	a membrane that separates the outer section of the ear from the middle and internal sections of the ear	鼓膜	鼓膜
ear infection (n)	an infection of the ear, usually causing inflammation and pain	耳部感染	耳部感染
ear wax (n)	the wax-like secretions of certain glands lining the canal of the outer ear	耳垢	耳垢
ear, nose, and throat (n)	a branch of medicine studying the ears, nose, and throat	耳鼻喉	耳鼻喉
ear, nose, and throat specialist (n)	a physician who specializes in the branch of medicine that combines treatment of the ear, nose, and throat	耳鼻喉專科醫生	耳鼻喉专科医生
earache (n)	an ache or pain in the ear	耳痛	耳痛
earlobe (n)	the fleshy bottom portion of the external ear	耳垂	耳垂
echocardiography (n)	a diagnostic technique utilizing ultrasound to visualize the internal structure of the heart	超聲波心動描記術	超声波心动描记术
eclampsia (n)	convulsions and coma occurring in a pregnant woman, associated with preeclampsia, i.e., hypertension and edema	子癇	子痫

English/Chinese Medical Glossary - E

ectopic pregnancy (n)	the development of a fetus outside the uterus	子宮外妊娠	子宫外妊娠
eczema (n)	a noncontiguous inflammation of the skin, marked mainly by redness, itching, and the outbreak of lesions that discharge matter and become encrusted and scaly	濕疹	湿疹
edema (n)	an excessive accumulation of fluid in tissue caused by diseases of the heart, kidney, liver, and veins	水腫	水肿
effect (n)	result produced by an action	效果	效果
effective (adj)	producing the intended result	有效的	有效的
effusion (n)	escape of fluid into a part of tissue	滲漏	渗漏
eggs (n)	1. the thin-shelled embryo of any bird, high in protein and cholesterol, and eaten alone or added to many foods including baked foods, breads, pasta, and packaged foods; 2. human egg cell	①蛋；②卵細胞	①蛋；②卵细胞
ejaculation (n)	a sudden act of expulsion; the sexual climax or orgasm in a male causing the release of semen	射精	射精
eject (v)	to throw out forcefully; to expel	排斥，射出	排斥，射出
elastic (adj)	capable of resisting and recovering from stretching, compression, or distortion applied by force	彈性的	弹性的
elbow (n)	the joint or bend of the arm between the forearm and the upper arm	肘	肘
elective (n)	subject to the choice or decision of the patient or physician; applied to procedures that are advantageous to the patient but not urgent	選擇	选择

English/Chinese Medical Glossary - E

English	Definition	Traditional	Simplified
electric stimulation (n)	transcutaneous electric nerve stimulation (TENS); therapy to reduce pain and restore muscle action	電刺激	电刺激
electrocardiogram (n)	a graph created by monitoring the electrical action of the heart; it is used to diagnose heart disease	心電圖	心电图
electrocardiograph (n)	an instrument used to record the potential of the electric currents that traverse the heart and initiate its contraction	心電圖描記器	心电图描记器
electroencephalography (n)	the recording of the electric currents developed in the brain, by means of electrodes applied to the scalp, to the surface of the brain, or placed within the substance of the brain; it is commonly used to diagnose seizures	腦電描記法	脑电描记法
electrolyte (n)	substance that dissociates into ions when in a solution, and is capable of conducting electricity	電解質	电解质
electromyelogram (n)	a graphic recording of muscle action	脊髓電圖	脊髓电图
elevator (n)	a platform or enclosure raised and lowered in a vertical shaft to transport things or people	電梯	电梯
elimination (n)	the act of removing; the excretion of waste from the body	排除	排除
elisa test (n)	enzyme-linked immunosorbent assay; a sensitive diagnostic test for measuring the amount of a substance (e.g., used in HIV testing)	酶免疫吸附劑測定	酶免疫吸附剂测定
embolism (n)	sudden blocking of an artery by a clot or foreign material	栓塞	栓塞
embryo (n)	the developing baby in the uterus from about two weeks after fertilization to the end of the seventh or eighth week	胚胎	胚胎

English/Chinese Medical Glossary - E

emergency (n)	an unexpected situation or sudden occurrence of a serious and urgent nature, usually life threatening, that demands immediate action	緊急	紧急
emergency room (n)	the section of the hospital where emergency cases are treated	急診室	急诊室
emergency services (n)	health services that are required for the alleviation of severe pain or immediate diagnosis and treatment of unforeseen medical conditions, which if not immediately diagnosed and treated, could lead to disability or death	緊急服務	紧急服务
emesis (n)	vomiting; an act of vomiting	嘔吐	呕吐
emetic (adj)	an agent that causes vomiting	催吐的	催吐的
emollient (n)	an agent that softens or soothes	潤滑劑	润滑剂
emotion (n)	a complex and usually strong feeling or response, such as love or fear	情緒	情绪
emotional (adj)	of, or pertaining to emotion	情緒的	情绪的
emphysema (n)	an accumulation of air in tissues or organs; applied especially to such a condition of the lungs	肺氣腫	肺气肿
empiric (adj)	depending upon experience or observation alone, without using a scientific method or theory	經驗嘗試的	经验尝试的
enamel (n)	the hard substance covering the exposed portion of a tooth	牙釉質，琺瑯質	牙釉质
encephalitis (n)	inflammation of the brain	腦炎	脑炎
encounter (n)	a medically related service or visit rendered by a provider to a beneficiary who is enrolled in a health plan on a specific date of service	出診	出诊

English/Chinese Medical Glossary - E

endemic (adj)	of, or pertaining to a disease present or usually prevalent in a population or geographical area at all times	地方性的	地方性的
endocrine system (n)	pertaining to the functioning and regulation of glands that secrete hormones throughout the body	內分泌系統	内分泌系统
endocrinologist (n)	a person whose profession is to study the physiology of the endocrine glands	內分泌學家	内分泌学家
endometriosis (n)	a condition in which endometrial-like tissue is found in the pelvic region	子宮內膜異位	子宫内膜异位
endometrium (n)	the membrane lining the uterus	子宮內膜	子宫内膜
endoscope (n)	an instrument for examining the interior of a bodily canal or hollow organ	內窺鏡	内窥镜
endoscopy (n)	visual inspection of any cavity of the body by using an endoscope	內窺鏡檢查	内窥镜检查
endotrachael intubation (n)	a surgical procedure that places a tube directly into the airway by way of the trachea to assist breathing	氣管內插管法	气管内插管法
endotracheal tube (n)	a tube inserted into the trachea to assist breathing	氣管內導管	气管内导管
enema (n)	an injection of liquid into the rectum through the anus for cleansing, as a laxative, or for other therapeutic purposes	灌腸	灌肠
energetic (adj)	exhibiting energy; strenuous; operating with force, vigor, or effect	精力充沛的	精力充沛的
energy (n)	the element a body requires to grow, develop, and work properly	能量	能量
environment (n)	sum total of all the conditions and elements which make up the surroundings of and influence the development and actions of an individual	環境	环境

English/Chinese Medical Glossary - E

enzyme (n)	a protein molecule that helps chemical reactions of other substances without itself being destroyed or altered upon completion of the reactions	酶	酶
epidemic (adj)	of, or pertaining to a disease that effects many people at the same time in the same geographic area	流行性的	流行性的
epidemiological (adj)	relating to, or involving the study of how diseases develop, spread, and affect populations	流行病學的	流行病学的
epidermal (adj)	of, or pertaining to, or resembling the outer, protective surface of skin, esp. a type of injection made into the skin	表皮的	表皮的
epidural (adj)	situated upon or outside the dura mater	硬膜外的	硬膜外的
epiglottis (n)	a small piece of cartilage that prevents food from entering the lungs when swallowing by covering the windpipe	會厭炎	会厌炎
epilepsy (n)	a disorder characterized by recurring attacks of motor, sensory, or psychic malfunction with or without unconsciousness or convulsive movements	癲癇	癫痫
epiphyseal (adj)	pertaining to or of the nature of a section of a bone, often an end of a long bone, that initially develops separated from the main portion by cartilage	骨骺的	骨骺的
episiotomy (n)	surgical incision into the region between the vagina and anus to prevent traumatic tearing during delivery of a baby	外陰切開術	外阴切开术

English/Chinese Medical Glossary - E

English	Definition	Traditional	Simplified
episode (n)	a noteworthy happening or series of happenings occurring in the course of continuous events, such as an episode of illness; a separate but related incident	發作	发作
epithelial (adj)	of, or pertaining to the epithelium	上皮的	上皮的
epithelium (n)	the layer of cells that form the surface lining of the mouth, digestive tract, and other mucous surfaces	上皮細胞	上皮细胞
equivalent (n)	having the same value; neutralizing or counterbalancing	等價物	等价物
erection (n)	condition of being made rigid and elevated, esp. the enlargement of the penis when aroused	勃起	勃起
erosion (n)	the destruction of the surface of a tissue, material, or structure	腐蝕	腐蚀
eruption (n)	act of breaking out, appearing, or becoming visible, as eruption of the teeth	長出，發疹	长出，发疹
erythema (n)	an area of skin which is red in color	紅斑	红斑
esophagitis (n)	inflammation of the esophagus or throat	食管炎	食管炎
esophagus (n)	a muscular membranous tube for the passage of food from the mouth to the stomach	食管	食管
estrogen (n)	any of several steroid hormones produced chiefly by the ovary and responsible for promoting the development and maintenance of female secondary sex characteristics	雌激素	雌激素
etiology (n)	study of the causes of disease	病因學	病因学
euphoria (n)	an exaggerated feeling of physical and mental well-being, especially when not justified by external reality	假欣快感	假欣快感

English/Chinese Medical Glossary - E

eustachian tube (n)	a bony and cartilaginous tube connecting the ear with the throat	耳喉管	耳喉管
evacuation (n)	an emptying, esp. of the bowels	排泄	排泄
evaluation (n)	the act or result of ascertaining or fixing the value or worth of; the act or result of examining or judging carefully	評價	评价
event monitor (n)	portable instrument used to monitor heart function	心電監測器	心电监测器
evolution (n)	process of development in which an organ or organism becomes more complex or changes due to pressures caused by the environment	進化	进化
exacerbation (n)	increase in the severity of a disease or its symptoms	加重	加重
exam (n) (m)	an examination or the act of observing, analyzing, questioning, and testing the state or condition of a person	檢查	检查
exam room (n)	the location where a doctor examines a patient	檢查室	检查室
excessive (adj)	exceeding the usual, proper, or normal quantity; more than necessary	過多的	过多的
excrete (v)	to eliminate waste from the blood, tissues, or organs	排泄	排泄
excretion (n)	the act, process, or function of eliminating waste from blood, tissue, or organs	排泄物	排泄物
exercise (n)	activity that requires physical or mental exertion, esp. when performed to develop or maintain fitness or good health	運動	运动
exercise tolerance test (n)	a method of measuring a person's level of physical condition	運動耐受試驗	运动耐受试验
exfoliation (n)	a falling off in scales or layers, esp. the loss of skin	脫落	脱落
exhale (v)	to breathe out	呼出	呼出

English/Chinese Medical Glossary - E

exit (n) (m)	a passage or way out	出口	出口
expectorant (n)	a drug/substance that promotes the ejection, by spitting, of mucus or other fluids from the lungs and throat	祛痰劑	祛痰剂
experimental (adj) (m)	of, or pertaining to, or based upon a test procedure, idea or activity	實驗性的	实验性的
expiration (n)	the act of breathing out, or expelling air from the lungs	斷氣	断气
exploratory surgery (n)	a surgical procedure used to investigate systematically a part of the body for the purpose of diagnosis	探查術	探查术
extend (v)	to straighten a leg or an arm	伸展	伸展
external use (n)	generally used in describing products such as ointments, salves, eye or ear drops that are not to be ingested	外用	外用
extract (v)	to separate a substance from something, esp. the removal of a desired substance from a plant or animal in order to prepare a drug	提取，萃取	提取，萃取
extraction (n)	the process or act of pulling or drawing out	提取，萃取	提取，萃取
extreme (adj)	as far away as possible from the center, the beginning or the average; of the highest degree or intensity	極度的；末端的	极度的；末端的
extremity (n)	a limb; an arm or leg; sometimes applied specifically to a hand or foot	端	端
eye (n)	an organ that allows humans to see and sense light	眼睛	眼睛
eye chart (n)	an instrument used to determine the quality of someone's vision	視力檢查表	视力检查表
eye drops (n)	a liquid medicine placed on the surface of the eye	滴眼劑	滴眼剂

English/Chinese Medical Glossary - E

eye exam (n)	a procedure where the physician studies the patient's eyes to detect any disease or vision problems	眼部檢查	眼部检查
eye patch (n)	a protective covering for the eye	眼罩	眼罩
eye strain (n)	over use of the muscles surrounding the eye characterized by pain in the eyes, tears, headache, or dizziness	視覺疲勞	视觉疲劳
eyeball (n)	the eye itself; the ball-shaped portion of the eye	眼球	眼球
eyebrows (n)	the bony ridge extending over the eye; the arch of short hairs covering this ridge	眉毛	眉毛
eyelash (n)	one of a row of short hairs at the edge of the eyelid	睫毛	睫毛
eyelid (n)	either of two folds of skin and muscle that can be closed over an eye	眼瞼	眼睑

Notes

English/Chinese Medical Glossary - F

face (n)	the surface of the front of the head from the top of the forehead to the base of the chin and from ear to ear	臉	脸
face-lift operation (n)	plastic surgery for tightening facial tissues and improving the appearance of facial skin	面部除皺術	面部除皱术
facial (adj)	of, or pertaining to the face	面部的	面部的
faint (v) (m)	to suddenly lose strength or vigor; to fall unconscious	昏倒	昏倒
faith (n)	firm and devoted adherence, as to a person, idea, or thing	信念	信念
fallopian tube (n)	either of a pair of slender ducts that connect the uterus to the ovaries in the female reproductive system	輸卵管	输卵管
family (n)	a group of persons sharing common ancestry	家人	家人
family doctor (n)	a physician who does not specialize in a particular area but treats a variety of medical problems, usually serving a family	家庭醫生	家庭医生
family nurse practitioner (n)	a nurse who is licensed to treat people of any age	家庭執業護理師	家庭执业护理师
family planning (n)	planning of the number of one's children through birth-control techniques	家庭計劃 計劃生育	家庭计划 计划生育
farsighted (n)	able to see objects better from a distance than from short range	遠視	远视
fast (v) (m)	to eat very little, nothing, or only select foods	禁食	禁食
fast foods (n)	any of various foods high in cholesterol, oils, and fats, including hamburgers, hotdogs, french fries, and pizza, and purchased at a grocery store or restaurant	方便食品，速食	方便食品，快餐

English/Chinese Medical Glossary - F

fat (n)	the main storage and source of energy in humans; a high energy nutrient found in butter, lard, grease, and oil, also found at high levels in meat, desserts, cheese, cream, and milk	脂肪	脂肪
fatal (adj)	causing death, deadly; mortal; lethal	致命的	致命的
fatigue (n)	a feeling of tiredness following exercise or strenuous activities	疲勞	疲劳
fats (n)	along with proteins and carbohydrates, on of the three nutrient groups used as energy sources by the body.	脂肪	脂肪
feces (n)	the substance discharged from the intestines, consisting of bacteria, cells, secretions (chiefly of the liver), and a small amount of undigested food	糞便	粪便
federal (n)	belonging to the central government of the United States	聯邦	联邦
Federal Financial Participation (n)	federal expenditures provided to match proper State expenditures made under State approved plans	聯邦政府的金融參與	联邦政府的金融参与
Federal Poverty Level (n)	poverty guidelines of the federal poverty measure. They are issued each year in the Federal Register by the Department of Health and Human Services (HHS). The guidelines are a simplification of the poverty thresholds for use for administrative purposes — for instance, determining financial eligibility for certain federal programs	聯邦政府的貧困標準	联邦政府的贫困标准
federally funded (n)	supported by monies from the Federal government	聯邦政府贊助	联邦政府赞助

© 2011 Cross Cultural Health Care Program

English/Chinese Medical Glossary - F

feedback (n)	the return of information about the result of a process, idea or activity	回饋	反馈
fee-for-service (n)	a method of reimbursement based on payment for specific services rendered to an enrollee. Payment may be made by an insurance carrier. Fee-for-service is the traditional method of reimbursement used by physicians and almost always occurs retrospectively (i.e. after the service has been rendered)	醫療費	医疗费
femur (n)	the bone in the leg that extends from the hip to the knee; the femur constitutes the upper leg, that part of the leg <u>above</u> the knee and is the largest bone in the human body	股骨	股骨
fertile (adj)	capable of reproducing	能生育的	能生育的
fertility (n)	the capacity to have a baby or to become pregnant	生育力	生育力
fester (v)	to generate pus	膿瘡	脓疱
fetal heart tone (n)	the heart beat of a fetus	胎兒心跳音	胎儿心跳音
fetal surgery (n)	any procedure that involves surgery on a fetus	胎兒外科	胎儿外科
fetus (n)	the unborn young of a human from the eighth week of pregnancy until birth	胎兒	胎儿
fever (n)	abnormally high body temperature, usually associated with illness	發燒	发烧
fiber (n) (m)	a slender, long structure; any of the elongated cells of muscle tissue; any of the filaments making up connective tissue	纖維絲	纤维丝
fiber (n) (m)	an important nutrient found in fruits, cereals, and grains	纖維	纤维
fibroid (n)	resembling or composed of fibrous tissue	纖維狀	纤维状

English/Chinese Medical Glossary - F

fibroid tumor (n)	a benign tumor of smooth muscle, esp. in the uterus	纖維瘤	纤维瘤
fibrous (adj)	of, pertaining to, or resembling fiber	纖維〈性〉的	纤维〈性〉的
fibula (n)	the outer and smaller of two bones of the leg between the knee and ankle	腓骨	腓骨
file (n)	a collection of information organized and easily retrievable, esp. a patient's history	文檔	文档
filling (n)	something used to fill a space, cavity, or container, such as a tooth filling	充填	充填
filtration (n)	passage of a liquid through a filter, accomplished by gravity, pressure, or vacuum suction	過濾	过滤
finger (n)	one of the five digits of the hand, esp. one other than the thumb	手指	手指
fingernail (n)	a thin, horny, transparent plate covering the surface of the tip of each finger	手指甲	手指甲
fingerprint (n)	the pattern on a surface left by the finger and used in identification	指紋	指纹
fingertips (n)	the end or distal section of the finger	指尖	指尖
fire extinguisher (n)	a portable or wheeled apparatus used for putting out small fires; it ejects extinguishing chemicals	滅火器	灭火器
first aid (n)	emergency treatment administered to injured or sick persons before professional medical care is available	急救	急救
fissure (n)	any cleft or groove, normal or otherwise, such as a fold in the cerebral cortex, skin, or mucous membrane	裂	裂

English/Chinese Medical Glossary - F

fistula (n)	an abnormal passage or communication, usually between two internal organs, or leading from an internal organ to the surface of the body	瘺道	瘘道
fixation (n) (m)	he act or operation of holding, suturing, or fastening in a fixed position	固定術	固定术
flaccid (adj)	weak, lax, and soft	弛緩的	弛缓的
flare-up (n)	a sudden outburst or intensification	突然發作	突然发作
flatulence (n)	presence of excessive amounts of air or gases in the stomach or intestine, leading to enlarging of the organs	氣脹	气胀
fleshy (adj)	similar or related to the soft tissue of the body, skin, or flesh; having a juicy or pulpy feeling	肉的	肉的
floaters (n)	black spots in front of the eyes caused by debris in the fluid inside the eye	懸浮物	悬浮物
floss (n)	a piece of waxed or unwaxed string used to remove plaque from below the gums and between the teeth	牙線	牙线
flu (n)	influenza; an acute infectious disease causing inflammation of the respiratory tract, fever, muscular pain, and irritation in the digestive system	流感	流感
fluoride (n)	a chemical compound used by dentists to help prevent tooth decay and disease	氯化物	氯化物
fluoroscopy (n)	a process using x-rays that allows continuous viewing of the internal structure of a human	螢光屏檢查	荧光屏检查

English/Chinese Medical Glossary - F

flush (v) (m)	to become red, esp. the skin on the face, usually from certain diseases, ingestion of certain drugs or other substances, heat, emotional factors, or physical exertion	潮紅	潮红
flutter (n)	a disturbance of normal heart rhythm	撲動	扑动
foam (n)	a mass of gas bubbles, esp. a light, bubbly gas and liquid mass formed by shaking a liquid containing certain soaps or detergents	泡沫	泡沫
follow-up (n)	the act or process of meeting again with a physician to reassess a person's health	隨訪	随访
fontanelle (n)	the soft portion of a baby's skull	囟門	囟门
Food and Drug Administration (n)	a federal consumer protection agency; its mission is to promote and protect public health by helping safe and effective products reach the market in a timely way, and monitoring products for continued safety after they are in use	食品與藥品管理局	食品与药品管理局
Food Guide Pyramid (n)	a graphic representation of guidelines developed to help people choose what to eat and how much to eat from the five basic food groups in order to get needed nutrients	食物指標金字塔	食物指标金字塔
food poisoning (n)	poisoning or illness caused by eating food contaminated by natural toxins or bacteria	食物中毒	食物中毒
foot (n)	the lower part of the leg that is in direct contact with the ground in standing or walking	腳	脚
forceps (n)	an instrument like a pair of tongs, used for grasping, manipulating, or extracting	鉗子	钳子
forearm (n)	the part of the arm between the elbow and the hand	前臂	前臂

English/Chinese Medical Glossary - F

forehead (n)	the part of the head or face between the eyebrows and the normal hairline	前額	前额
foreskin (n)	the excess of skin covering the end of the penis	包皮	包皮
fortified (n)	strengthened or reinforced	強化	强化
fraction (n)	a small part; bit; a substance separated from another	部分	部分
fracture (n)	a break or rupture in a bone	骨折	骨折
freckle (n)	a small spot of coloring in the skin, often brought out by the sun	雀斑	雀斑
frequency (n) (m)	number of occurrences of a periodic or recurrent process per unit of time	頻率	频率
fried food (n)	any of various foods cooked in oil and high in fats and cholesterol, including french fries, fried chicken, or fried fish	油炸食品	油炸食品
fright (n)	sudden, intense fear, as of something immediately threatening, alarming, or strange	驚嚇	惊吓
frighten (v)	to make afraid; to alarm	使驚嚇	使惊吓
front desk (n)	a location in a building used to greet people as they enter, manned/serviced by a desk clerk	服務台	服务台
frostbite (n)	local tissue destruction resulting from freezing, esp. damaged skin of the fingers and toes	凍瘡	冻疮
frozen shoulder (n)	a shoulder that cannot be moved	凍肩，肩動困難	冻肩，肩动困难
fruit (n)	a sweet and fleshy part of a plant, served as food, such as oranges, apples, grapes, plums, and bananas	果實	果实
fruit juices (n)	any of various beverages made from the liquid of a fruit	果汁	果汁
function (n) (m)	the special, normal, or proper activity of an organ or part	功能	功能

English/Chinese Medical Glossary - F

fundamental (adj)	of, or pertaining to a base or foundation, esp. the foundation of an idea	基本的	基本的
funeral home (n)	an establishment in which the dead are prepared for burial or cremation, and in which wakes and funerals may be held	殯儀館	殡仪馆
fungicide (n)	an agent that destroys fungi	殺真菌劑	杀真菌剂
fungus (n)	general term used to denote a group of cellular organisms including mushrooms, yeasts, rusts, molds, smuts, etc.	真菌	真菌

Notes

English/Chinese Medical Glossary - G

gait (n)	manner or style of walking	步態	步态
gallbladder (n)	a small pear-shaped muscular sac located under the liver, in which bile secreted by the liver is stored	膽囊	胆囊
gallstone (n)	a small, hard mass formed in the gallbladder or in a bile duct	膽石	胆石
ganglion (n)	a group of nerve cells found outside of the brain or spinal cord	神經節	神经节
gangrene (n)	the death and decay of tissue, usually caused by infection, injury, or lack of blood supply to the tissue	壞疽	坏疽
gargle (v)	to force exhaled air through a liquid held in the back of the mouth in order to cleanse or medicate the mouth or throat	漱口	漱口
gas (n)	the state of matter distinguished from solid and liquid states by very low density (e.g., air that passes through the intestine, air inhaled for anesthesia) and the ability to diffuse readily	氣	气
gastric (adj)	of, or pertaining to the stomach	胃部的	胃部的
gastric bleeding (n)	bleeding in the stomach	胃出血	胃出血
gastric juice (n)	secretions in the stomach that assist in digestion	胃液	胃液
gastric ulcer (n)	an ulcer located in the stomach	胃潰瘍	胃溃疡
gastritis (n)	inflammation of the stomach	胃炎	胃炎
gastroenteritis (n)	an acute inflammation of the lining of the stomach and intestines, characterized by nausea, diarrhea, abdominal pain, and weakness, which has various causes, including food poisoning and infection	胃腸炎	胃肠炎
gastroenterologist (n)	person who specializes in diseases of the digestive tract	胃腸病醫生	胃肠病医生

English/Chinese Medical Glossary - G

Gastroesophageal Reflux Disease (GERD) (n)	a condition wherein acidic stomach contents regurgitate or back up (reflux) into the esophagus, causing inflammation and damage to the esophagus; this frequently causes heartburn because of irritation of the esophagus by stomach acid	胃食道逆流疾病	胃食道逆流疾病
gastrointestinal (adj)	of, or pertaining to, or communication with the stomach and intestine	胃腸的	胃肠的
gatekeeper (n)	the term used in a managed care plan to refer to the physician who has primary responsibility for providing basic medical services and coordinating a patient's medical care and referrals; in order for a patient to receive specialty referrals or a hospital admission, the gatekeeper must typically authorize it, unless there is an emergency	看門人	看门人
gauze (n)	a thin, transparent fabric with a loose open weave, used for covering wounds	紗布	纱布
gene (n)	a functional hereditary unit that occupies a fixed location on a chromosome, has a specific influence on the phenotype, and is capable of mutating	基因	基因
general anesthesia (n)	the use of drugs to cause a person to lose all sense of feeling, thus enabling painless surgery	全身麻醉	全身麻醉
general practitioner (n)	a physician who does not specialize in a particular area but treats a variety of medical problems	全科醫師	全科医师
genetic (adj)	of, or pertaining to genes, reproduction, or to birth	遺傳的	遗传的

English/Chinese Medical Glossary - G

genetic counseling (n)	the counseling of prospective parents on the probabilities of inherited diseases occurring in offspring and on the diagnosis and treatment of such diseases	遺傳諮詢	遗传咨询
genetic factors (n)	biological information (genes, characteristics) that parents pass on to their children	遺傳因素	遗传因素
genetic tendency (n)	susceptibility to a particular disease due to genetics	遺傳趨勢	遗传趋势
genital (adj)	of, or relating to reproduction; of, or pertaining to the genitalia	生殖器的	生殖器的
genitalia (n)	the reproductive organs, esp. the external sexual organs	生殖器	生殖器
geriatric (n)	associated with the elderly	老年醫學	老年医学
germ (n) (m)	pathogenic microorganism; something that may serve as the basis of further growth or development	胚芽，細菌	胚芽，细菌
German Measles (n)	a mild, contagious, eruptive disease with widespread pink rash caused by a virus and capable of causing defects in infants born to mothers infected during the first three months of pregnancy (i.e., rubella)	風疹	风疹
gestation (n)	period of development of the young, from the time of fertilization of the ovum until birth	妊娠	妊娠
gestational diabetes (n)	a specific form of diabetes caused by pregnancy	妊娠糖尿病	妊娠糖尿病
gingivitis (n)	inflammation of the gums	齒齦炎	齿龈炎
give a shot (v)	to inject medicine under a person's skin	打針	打针
gland (n)	an organ that extracts specific substances from the blood and concentrates or alters them for subsequent secretion	腺	腺

English/Chinese Medical Glossary - G

glandular (adj)	of, or pertaining to, or resembling a gland or the activities of a gland	腺的	腺的
glans penis (n)	the end of the penis	陰莖頭	阴茎头
glasses (eye) (n)	a pair of lenses mounted in a light frame, used to correct poor vision or to protect the eyes	眼鏡	眼镜
glaucoma (n)	a disease of the eye characterized by an increase in pressure in the eye, which causes defects in vision	青光眼	青光眼
glottis (n)	the space between the vocal chords at the upper part of the larynx or voice box	聲門	声门
glucometer (n)	a device that measures the amount of sugar in a human's blood	血糖儀	血糖仪
glucose (n)	sugar found in certain foods, especially fruits, and in the normal blood of all animals; a major source of energy for humans, also see *carbohydrate*	葡萄糖	葡萄糖
gluten (n)	protein of wheat and other grains	麩質	麸质
goiter (n)	a chronic enlargement of the thyroid gland, visible as swelling at the front of the neck, associated with iodine deficiency	甲狀腺腫	甲状腺肿
gonad (n)	an organ involved in reproduction, i.e., the testis or ovaries	生殖腺	生殖腺
gonorrhea (n)	sexually transmitted infection; male may experience pain and discharge from the penis; female may be asymptomatic or have vaginal discharge	淋病	淋病

English/Chinese Medical Glossary - G

gout (n)	a disturbance of the metabolic system occurring predominantly in males, characterized by painful inflammation of the joints, esp. of the feet and hands	痛風	痛风
gown (hospital) (n)	a loose garment worn by patients in the hospital	罩衣	罩衣
gradual (adj)	taking place by a series of small changes over a long period; not sudden	逐漸的	逐渐的
grains (n)	any of various small hard seeds used in making bread or cereal and high in fiber and carbohydrates	穀粒	谷粒
Graves Disease (n)	a disease causing a toxic goiter	格雷夫斯病	格雷夫斯病
gravidity (n)	pregnancy; the condition of being pregnant, without regard to the outcome	妊娠	妊娠
grievance (n)	1) a written request by a provider for a health plan to review an adverse action decision, or policy issued by the health plan which has a direct effect on the provider; and 2) a written request by a member for a health plan to review an action or decision by the health plan or one of its providers	申訴	申诉
groin (n)	the area of the body found between the legs and at the junction between the trunk and legs, including the external genitals	腹股溝	腹股沟
guardian (n)	person charged with the care of the person or property of another	監護人	监护人

English/Chinese Medical Glossary - G

gums (n)	that part of the lining of the oral cavity (oral mucosa) that surrounds the base of the teeth generally red or pink in color; it may be the site of injury, inflammation, bleeding or infection; often a concern if the gums are receding, starting to cover less and less of a tooth or a series of teeth	牙齦	牙龈
gun shot wound (n)	any injury resulting from a bullet	射擊傷	射击伤
gynecological (adj)	of, or pertaining to gynecology	婦科的	妇科的
gynecology (n)	the medical science of disease, reproductive physiology, and endocrinology in women	婦科	妇科
Gynecologist (n)	a person who studies diseases, disorders, and physiology of the female reproductive organs	婦科學家	妇科学家

Notes

English/Chinese Medical Glossary - H

habitual (adj)	the nature of a habit; according to habit; something done repeatedly without thinking	習慣的	习惯的
Haemophilus Influenza Type B (HiB) (n)	a bacteria capable of causing a range of diseases including ear infections, cellulitis (soft tissue infection), upper respiratory infections, pneumonia, and such serious "invasive" infections as meningitis with potential brain damage and epiglottitis with airway obstruction; more than 90% of all HIB infections occur in children 5 years of age or less; the peak attack rate is at 6-12 months of age	B型流行感冒嗜血桿菌 (HiB)	B型流感嗜血杆菌 (HiB)
hair (n)	one of the cylindrical, often colored filaments growing from the skin of a human	頭髮	头发
hairline (n)	the edge of a person's hair, esp. along the top of the forehead	頭髮輪廓線	头发轮廓线
halitosis (n)	a foul odor from the mouth	口臭	口臭
hallucination (n)	false or distorted perception of objects or events with a compelling sense of reality, usually as a product of mental disorder or as a response to a drug	幻覺	幻觉
hand (n) (m)	the end of the human arm below the wrist, consisting of the palm, four fingers, and a thumb	手	手
handicapped (adj)	at a disadvantage or suffering from a deficiency, esp. a physical or mental disability that prevents or restricts normal activities	殘疾的	残疾的
hangover (n)	unpleasant feeling or sensation following the heavy or over use of alcohol	宿醉	宿醉

English/Chinese Medical Glossary - H

Hansen's disease (n)	leprosy; a chronic, infectious disease that causes lumps on the skin	漢森氏病	汉森氏病
hardening of the arteries (n)	a condition in which excess cholesterol builds up inside the arteries, causing them to narrow; also referred to as "atherosclerosis"	動脈硬化	动脉硬化
hay fever, allergic rhinitis (n)	an acute allergic condition of the eyes and respiratory system, characterized by a running nose, sneezing, and headaches, and often caused by an abnormal sensitivity to certain airborne pollens	花粉症，過敏性鼻炎	花粉症，过敏性鼻炎
head (n)	the uppermost part of the body, containing the brain, ears, eyes, mouth, and jaw	頭	头
headache (n)	a pain in the head	頭痛	头痛
heal (v)	to restore to health or soundness; to cure	痊癒	痊愈
health (n)	the overall condition of a person at any given time	健康	健康
health care (n)	the prevention, treatment, and management of illness and the preservation of mental and physical well-being through the services offered by the medical and health professions	健康照護	健康照护
Health Care Agency (n)	a local administrative entity responsible for providing public and preventive health services to the citizens	健康照護機構	健康照护机构
Health Care Financing Administration (HCFA) (n)	The federal agency responsible for administering Medicare and overseeing State administration of Medicaid. HCFA is now known as CMS – Center for Medicaid & State Operations	健康照護資金管理局	健康照护资金管理局

English/Chinese Medical Glossary - H

health care provider (n)	a person or institution (i.e. doctor, nurse, hospital, insurance company, health maintenance organization) that provides health care services to people	健康照護提供者	健康照护提供者
health care services (n)	services provided with the purpose of taking care of the health of individuals	健康照護服務	健康照护服务
Health Consumer Action Center (HCAC) (n)	an advocy group working to protect the rights of consumers	健康消費者行動中心	健康消费者行动中心
health educator (n)	a practitioner who is professionally prepared in the field of health education, who demonstrates competence in both theory and practice, and who accepts responsibility to advance the aims of the health education profession	健康教育工作者	健康教育工作者
Health Insuring Organization (HIO) (n)	A local, public agency which receives all Medicaid funding that would be spent on eligibles in its area: arranges for the provision of all necessary medical services; and pays providers for those services	健康投保組織 (HIO)	健康投保组织 (HIO)
Health Maintenance Organization (HMO) (n)	an entity that provides, offers or arranges for coverage of designated health services needed by plan members for a fixed, prepaid premium. There are four basis models of HMOs: staff model, group model, network model and individual practice association	健康維護組織 (HMO)	健康维护组织 (HMO)
health network (n)	a group of health care professionals working with a hospital to provide services to patients under a contract with a health plan	健康網路	健康网络
Healthy Families Program (HFP) (n)	a state and federal funded health coverage program for children under the age of 19	健康家庭計劃	健康家庭计划

English/Chinese Medical Glossary - H

hear (v)	to perceive by the ear; to listen	聽	听
hearing aid (n)	an instrument placed in the ear to increase the sound level for a person who hears poorly	助聽器	助听器
hearing loss (n)	a condition of not being able to hear or sense sound; reduction in the ability to hear	聽覺喪失	听觉丧失
heart (n)	the hollow, muscular organ that pumps blood from veins to arteries and provides blood to the entire body	心	心
heart attack (n)	myocardial infarction or death of an area of heart muscle from lack of blood reaching the muscle, often due to coronary artery disease	心肌梗死，心臟病發作	心肌梗死，心脏病发作
heart defects (n)	any of numerous conditions where the heart does not function properly	心臟缺損	心脏缺损
heart disease (n)	occurs when blood vessels supplying blood to the heart muscle (the coronary arteries) are narrowed or blocked; the narrowing or blockage is most often caused by buildup of fat (cholesterol) and calcium inside the heart arteries	心臟病	心脏病
heart failure (n)	the inability of the heart to pump blood	心力衰竭	心力衰竭
heart murmur (n)	noise, heard usually with a stethoscope, that is caused by turbulent blood flow in the heart; may be normal or associated with heart or valvular disease	心雜音	心杂音
heart rate (n)	the number of heart beats per unit of time, usually per minute	心率	心率
heart trouble (n)	any difficulty, distress, disease, malfunction, etc., of the heart	心臟病	心脏病

English/Chinese Medical Glossary - H

heart valve (n)	one of several openings in the heart that controls the flow of blood into other chambers or areas of the heart	心瓣膜	心瓣膜
heartbeat (n)	a single contraction of the heart	心跳	心跳
heartburn (n)	a burning sensation caused by stomach acids backing up into the lower esophagus (the tube that leads from the mouth to the stomach); the acids produce a burning sensation and discomfort between the ribs just below the breast bone	胃灼熱，心口灼熱	胃灼热，燒心
heat (n)	a sensation of feeling hot; the condition of being hot	熱	热
heat exhaustion (n)	a reaction to excessive heat, marked by weakness and collapse resulting from a lack of water	中暑衰竭	中暑衰竭
heat stroke (n)	a severe illness caused by exposure to excessively high temperatures and characterized by severe headache, high fever, dry hot skin, and, in serious cases, collapse and coma	中暑	中暑
heel (n)	the rounded end portion of the foot under and behind the ankle	腳後跟(n)	脚后跟(n)
height (n)	a measurement of how tall someone is; stature, esp. of the human body	身高	身高
hematological (adj)	relating to hematology, the branch of medical science which treats diseases of the blood and blood-forming tissues	血液的	血液的
hematologist (n)	a person who specializes in the science encompassing the generation, anatomy, physiology, pathology, and therapeutics of blood	血液學家	血液学家

English/Chinese Medical Glossary - H

hematology (n)	the scientific study of the generation, anatomy, physiology, pathology, and therapeutics of blood	血液學	血液学
hematoma (n)	a localized collection of blood, usually clotted, in an organ, space, or tissue, due to a break in the wall of a blood vessel	血腫	血肿
hemiplegia (n)	paralysis of one side of the body, sometimes caused by a stroke	單側癱瘓	單側瘫痪
hemodialysis (n)	a filtration process to remove toxic substances from the blood in cases of kidney disorders	血液透析	血液透析
hemoglobin (n)	a protein found in red blood cells that carries oxygen	血紅蛋白	血红蛋白
hemophilia (n)	a hereditary condition characterized by the inability to stop bleeding	血友病	血友病
hemopoietic system (n)	the system of tissues and organs, including bone marrow, that are responsible for the production and development of blood cells	造血系統	造血系统
hemorrhage (n)	escape of blood from the vessels; bleeding	出血	出血
hemorrhoids (n)	an itching or painful mass of swollen veins at the anus	痔	痔
hepatic (adj)	of, or pertaining to the liver	肝的	肝的
hepatitis (n)	inflammation of the liver	肝炎	肝炎
Hepatitis A (n)	inflammation of the liver caused by the hepatitis A virus (HAV), which is usually transmitted by food or drink that has been handled by an infected person whose hygiene is poor; symptoms include nausea, fever, and jaundice (yellowing of the skin and/or eyes)	甲型肝炎	甲型肝炎

English/Chinese Medical Glossary - H

Hepatitis B (n)	inflammation of the liver due to the hepatitis B virus (HBV) once thought to be passed only through blood products; it is now known that hepatitis B can also be transmitted via needle sticks, body piercing, and tattooing using unsterilized instruments, the dialysis process, sexual and even less intimate close contact, and childbirth; symptoms include fatigue, jaundice, nausea, vomiting, dark urine, and light stools	乙型肝炎	乙型肝炎
herb (n)	a plant that has a fleshy stem, as distinguished from the woody tissue of shrubs and trees, and that generally dies back at the end of each growing season; any of various plants that smell, esp. in medicine	草藥	草药
herbalist (n)	one versed in herbal lore and, in regard to therapy, an herb doctor	草藥醫生	草药医生
hereditary (adj.)	derived or transmitted from an ancestor or parent, esp. referring to a disorder or disease	遺傳的	遗传的
heredity (n)	genetic transmission of a particular quality or trait from parent to offspring	遺傳	遗传
hermetic (adj)	completely sealed, esp. against the escape or entry of air	密封的	密封的
hernia (n)	protrusion of a loop or knuckle of an organ or tissue through an abnormal opening	疝氣	疝气
herniated disk (n)	the dislocation of cartilage found between two vertebrae in the spinal cord or back bone	椎間盤突出	椎间盘突出

English/Chinese Medical Glossary - H

herpes (n)	an inflammatory skin disease caused by the herpes virus, characterized by the eruption of blisters on the skin	皰疹	疱疹
herpes sore, cold sore, fever blister (n)	a painful eruption or blister on the skin caused by a herpes (HSV 1) infection	皰疹瘡，感冒瘡，發熱性皰疹	疱疹疮，感冒疮，发热性疱疹
hiccup (n)	a spasm of the diaphragm resulting in a sudden inhalation that is stopped by a rapid closing of the airway to the lungs	呃逆，打嗝	呃逆，打嗝
high blood pressure (n)	an increased or abnormally high level of pressure in the arteries	高血壓	高血压
hip (n)	the body part that projects sideways from the pelvis or pelvic region between the waist to the thigh	臀部	臀部
histology (n)	the study of the physical structure of tissue	組織學	组织学
history (medical) (n) (m)	a narrative of events; story; a chronological record of events, often including an explanation of or commentary on those events, esp. a record of a patient's medical background	病歷	病历
HIV (n)	acronym for the Human Immunodeficiency Virus, the cause of AIDS (acquired immunodeficiency syndrome)	人體免疫缺陷病毒 (HIV)	人体免疫缺陷病毒 (HIV)
hives (n)	a skin condition characterized by intensely itching welts and caused by allergic reactions to internal or external agents	蕁麻疹	荨麻疹
hoarse (adj)	having a husky and grating voice	聲嘶的	声嘶的
hobby (n)	a fun pastime	嗜好	嗜好
hold on (v)	to grasp or squeeze an object	抓住	抓住
hold your breath (v)	to refrain from expelling air from the lungs for a period of time	屏息	屏息

English/Chinese Medical Glossary - H

holter monitor (n)	small portable ECG device for long-term recording of electrical activity of the heart; may detect fleeting changes that might otherwise go unnoticed	動態心電圖監視器	动态心电图 监视器
home maker chores (n)	household services, including household cleaning, laundry, shopping, food preparation, and household maintenance	家務	家务
hormone (n)	a chemical substance produced in the body that controls and regulates the activity of certain cells or organs	荷爾蒙	荷尔蒙
hormone replacement therapy (n)	a combination therapy of estrogen plus progesterone, used to treat menopause	荷爾蒙替代療法	荷尔蒙替代疗法
hormone therapy (n)	a process of treating a disease with medication containing specific hormones	荷爾蒙治療	荷尔蒙治疗
hospice (n)	an establishment or a program that provides for the physical and emotional needs of terminally ill patients	安寧服務，姑息治療	安宁服务，姑息治疗
hospital (n)	an institution that provides medical or surgical care and treatment for the sick and the injured	醫院	医院
hospitalization (n)	confinement of a patient in a hospital, or the period of such confinement	住院治療	住院治疗
hot flashes (n)	a passing symptom of menopause that involves the sensation of heat all over the body	熱潮紅	热潮红
hot pack (n)	a sac or pouch that becomes warm from an internal chemical reaction and is placed on the skin to promote blood circulation	熱敷法	热敷法
hot water bottle (n)	a rubber container filled with hot water used to warm the bed or parts of the body	熱水瓶	热水瓶

English/Chinese Medical Glossary - H

humerus (n)	the long bone of the upper arm	肱骨	肱骨
humor (n) (m)	sense of finding things funny or amusing	液，體液	液，体液
hurt (v)	to cause physical damage or pain; to injure	損傷，疼痛	损伤，疼痛
hydration (n)	condition of being combined with water	水合作用	水合作用
hydrocephalus (n)	a condition in which an abnormal accumulation of fluid in the brain causes enlargement of the skull and compression of the brain	腦積水	脑积水
hydrogen peroxide (n)	a colorless, heavy, liquid used principally to clean wounds and medical equipment	過氧化氫	过氧化氢
hygiene (n)	prevention of disease through cleanliness	衛生	卫生
hymen (n)	a fold of tissue partly or completely blocking the opening of the vagina; normal, not pathologic	處女膜	处女膜
hyperactivity (n)	the state of being excessively active, moving more than normal	活動過度	活动过度
hyperglycemia (n)	a condition of a high level of sugar in the blood; see related words including *sugar, glucose,* and *carbohydrate*	血糖過多	血糖过多
hyperopia (n)	a condition in which the eye does not focus properly on objects at close range without the assistance of glasses; farsightedness	遠視	远视
hypertension (n)	continuously high blood pressure	高血壓	高血压
hyperthermia (n)	abnormally high body temperature, especially that induced for therapeutic purposes	高熱	高热
hyperthyroidism (n)	excessive functional activity of the thyroid gland; overproduction of thyroid hormone; opposite of hypothyroidism	甲狀腺機能亢進	甲状腺机能亢进

English/Chinese Medical Glossary - H

English	Definition	Traditional	Simplified
hyperventilation (n)	a state in which there is an increased amount of air entering the lungs	換氣過度	换气过度
hypnosis (n)	an induced sleeplike condition in which an individual is extremely responsive to suggestions made by the person causing this condition	催眠狀態	催眠状态
hypnotize (v)	to put in a state of hypnosis	催眠	催眠
hypochondriasis (n)	the continued belief that one is or is likely to become ill, often involving experiences of real pain, when illness is neither present nor likely	疑病症	疑病症
hypodermic (adj)	applied or administered beneath the skin	皮下的	皮下的
hypoglycemia (n)	a low level of sugar in the blood; see related words including *sugar, glucose,* and *carbohydrate*	低血糖	低血糖
hypothermia (n)	a low body temperature, as that due to exposure in cold weather or induced as a means of decreasing metabolism as used in various surgical procedures	低溫	低温
hypothyroidism (n)	reduction of thyroid activity, esp. the release of hormones	甲狀腺機能減退	甲状腺机能减退
hysterectomy (n)	operation of removing the uterus, and sometimes, ovaries, performed either through the abdominal wall or through the vagina	子宮切除術	子宫切除术

Notes

English/Chinese Medical Glossary - H

English/Chinese Medical Glossary - I

iatrogenic (adj)	resulting from the activity of physicians	醫源性的	医源性的
ICD-9 Codes/Coding System (n)	International Classification of Diseases (ICD-9) is a universally accpeted standard coding system utilized by healthcare providers	編號/編碼系統	编号/编码系统
ice pack (n)	a cold instrument used to cool the body and reduce the blood supply to an area	冰裹法	冰裹法
idiosyncrasy (n)	an abnormal sensitivity to some drug, protein, or other agent	特異反應，特異體質	特异反應，特异体质
ileum (n)	the last portion of the small intestine	迴腸	迴肠
immaturity (n)	state or quality of being not fully developed	未成熟	未成熟
immobilization (n)	act of rendering not movable, as by a cast or splint	制動，固定	制动，固定
immune (adj)	protected against infectious disease	免疫的	免疫的
immune system (n)	the activity, organs, glands, and structures in the body responsible for providing protection against disease	免疫系統	免疫系统
immunity (n)	protection against infectious disease	免疫	免疫
immunization (n)	the process of making someone immune to a disease, usually by injection of some substance	免疫法	免疫法
immunization schedule (n)	a calendar of recommended shots	免疫程序表	免疫程序表
immunize (v)	to render immune by injection (or oral medication)	使免疫	使免疫
immunology (n)	the medical study of the immune system and how it protects the body against infectious disease	免疫學	免疫学
impaired (adj)	reduced in strength, value, quantity, or quality	受損的	受损的
impaired vision (n)	the inability to see clearly	受損的視力	受损的视力

English/Chinese Medical Glossary - I

impetigo (n)	a skin infection caused by a specific bacteria characterized by blisters that erupt and form yellow crusts	膿皰病	脓疱病
implant (n) (m)	something implanted, esp. surgically implanted tissue	植入物	植入物
implant (v) (m)	to insert or embed surgically	植入	植入
implantation (n)	insertion or grafting into the body of biological, living, inert, or radioactive material	植入法	植入法
implication (n)	a possible effect of an action	牽連	牵连
impotence (n)	the condition of not being able to perform sexual intercourse, inability to get or maintain an erect penis	陽痿	阳痿
impregnation (n)	the act of rendering pregnant	受孕，受精	受孕，受精
In Home Supportive Services (IHSS) (n)	social or medical services provided in one's home	居家支援服務	居家支援服务
in situ (adj/adv)	in the original place; may refer to the origin of a cancerous tumor	原位	原位
in vitro (adv)	within a glass; observable in a test tube; in an artificial environment	在試管內	在试管内
inactive (adj)	not active; being out of use	不活躍的	不活跃的
incarceration (n) (m)	abnormal retention or confinement of a body part	禁閉	禁闭
incision (n)	a surgical cut into soft tissue; the act of cutting into or marking with a sharp instrument	切口	切口
incisor (n)	a tooth adapted for cutting, located at the front of the mouth	切牙，門牙	切牙，门牙
incompetence (n)	physical or mental inadequacy or insufficiency	機能不全	机能不全
incontinence (n)	inability to control excretory functions, as defecation or urination	失禁	失禁
incubation (n)	giving proper conditions for development	孵育	孵育

English/Chinese Medical Glossary - I

incubation period (n)	the length of time required for symptoms to be visible after entrance of a disease into the body	孵育期	孵育期
incubator (n)	a cabinet in which a uniform temperature can be maintained, used in growing bacteria, or in keeping small babies warm	孵化器，保溫箱	孵化器，保溫箱
index finger (n)	the finger next to the thumb	食指	食指
indication (n)	a sign or circumstance which points to or shows the cause, pathology, issue, or an attack of a disease	指示	指示
indigestion (n)	inability to eat or digest something, esp. food; discomfort or illness resulting from indigestion	消化不良	消化不良
induce (v)	to cause something to happen, esp. by the administration of medication	誘導	诱导
induced abortion (n)	a procedure or drug that causes an abortion	人工流產	人工流产
induced labor (n)	the act or process of causing a woman to begin the birthing of a child through medication or other medical procedure	引產，導產	引产，导產
induced vomiting (n)	a procedure or drug that causes vomiting	誘發嘔吐	诱发呕吐
infantile (adj)	pertaining to an infant or to infancy	嬰兒的	婴儿的
infantile paralysis (n)	poliomyelitis; an infectious viral disease occurring mainly in children and in its acute form attacking the central nervous system and producing paralysis	嬰兒麻痺	婴儿麻痹
infarct (n)	the death of tissue caused by a lack of blood to the tissue	梗塞	梗塞
infect (v)	to have microorganisms enter the body and produce harmful toxins	傳染	传染
infected (adj)	of, or pertaining to a person who has a disease	被感染的	被感染的

English/Chinese Medical Glossary - I

infection (n)	the invasion and multiplication of microorganisms in tissues	傳染	传染
infectious disease (n)	germs that invade the body and create an infection that can spread from person to person	傳染病	传染病
infertility (n)	the inability to reproduce	不育症	不育症
infiltration (n) (m)	the accumulation of a substance in a tissue or cell	浸潤	浸润
inflammation (n)	localized heat, redness, swelling, and pain as a result of irritation, injury, or infection	炎症	炎症
influenza (n)	acute viral infection involving the respiratory tract	流感	流感
informed consent (n)	the process of informing, educating, or telling a patient about a medical treatment, and obtaining the permission for the treatment from the patient	知情同意	知情同意
infuse (v)	to pour a liquid into something	注入	注入
infusion (n)	therapeutic introduction of a fluid other than blood, as saline solution, into a vein	注入物	注入物
ingestion (n)	the act of taking food, medicine, etc., into the body, by mouth	食入	食入
ingrown toenail (n)	a toenail that has grown into the skin causing inflammation	嵌趾甲	嵌趾甲
inguinal (adj)	of, or relating to, or located between the legs, or in the crease between the legs and the trunk	腹股溝的	腹股沟的
inhalation (n)	drawing of air or other substances into the lungs	吸入	吸入
inhale (v)	to draw in by breathing	吸入	吸入
inhaler (n)	a device that produces a vapor to ease breathing or to medicate by inspiration	吸入器	吸入器

English/Chinese Medical Glossary - I

injection (n)	forcing a liquid into a part, as into the skin, a vein, or an organ, by a needle	注射	注射
injure (v)	to cause harm to; to hurt	損傷	损伤
injured (adj)	pertaining to someone who sustained an injury	受傷的	受伤的
injury (n)	damage of or to a person, property, or thing	受傷處	受伤处
inner ear (n)	the portion of the ear that senses position for balance	內耳	內耳
inoculate (v)	to inject a substance into a person to produce an immunity against a disease	預防注射	预防注射
inorganic (adj)	not of organic origin; not of living matter	無機的	无机的
inpatient (n)	a patient staying in a medical facility for treatment	住院病人	住院病人
in-patient (n)	receiving services as a patient of a medical facility	住院	住院
insane (adj)	exhibiting, or afflicted with insanity	神經錯亂的	神经错乱的
insanity (n)	persistent mental disorder	精神病	精神病
insect bite (n)	the mark left on the skin from the bite of an insect	蟲咬	虫咬
insecticide (n)	a substance, chemical, or agent that kills insects	殺蟲劑	杀虫剂
insert (v)	to introduce into the body; to place inside	插入	插入
insertion (n)	place of attachment, as of a muscle to the bone which it moves	插入物	插入物
insidious (adj)	of, or pertaining to a disease that develops without symptoms	潛伏的，隱藏的	潜伏的，隐袭的
insomnia (n)	inability to sleep; abnormal wakefulness	失眠症	失眠症
inspiration (n)	act of drawing air into the lungs	吸氣	吸气
instability (n)	quality or state of being unstable or without balance	不穩定性	不稳定性
instep (n)	the arched portion of the foot	腳背	脚背
insulin (n)	a hormone that controls the level of sugar in the blood	胰島素	胰岛素

English/Chinese Medical Glossary - I

insulin reaction or shock (n)	low level of sugar in the blood caused by excessive insulin	胰島素反應/休克	胰岛素反应/休克
insult (n)	injury or trauma; attack, harmful action	發作，損傷	发作，损伤
insurance (n)	coverage by a contract binding a party to pay for loss of another party, esp. insurance that covers medical expenses	保險	保险
insurance company (n)	a business that sells insurance	保險公司	保险公司
intact (adj)	the condition of having something functional, complete, and living; having no relevant component removed or destroyed	完整的	完整的
intensive care (n)	special medical equipment and services provided for seriously ill patients; a hospital unit that specializes in intensive care	重症監護，加護病房	重症监护，重症监护病房
interaction (n)	quality, state, or process of two or more things acting on each other	交互作用	交互作用
intercourse (n)	1. dealings or communications between persons or groups; 2. sexual intercourse	①交流；②性交	①交流；②性交
intermediary (adj)	performed or occurring in a middle stage; neither early or late; intermediate	中間的	中间的
intermittent (adj)	occurring at separated intervals; having periods of lacking activity	間歇的	间歇的
internal (adj)	situated or occurring within or on the inside	內部的	内部的
internal bleeding (n)	the abnormal loss of blood into a cavity inside the body	內出血	内出血
internal medicine (n)	a medical specialty dedicated to the prevention, diagnosis, and treatment of diseases of adults	內科	内科
internist (n)	a physician who specializes in internal medicine, the medical study and treatment of non-surgical diseases in adults	內科醫師	内科医师

English/Chinese Medical Glossary - I

interpretation (n)	the act, process, or result of interpreting from one language to another in order to convey the meaning of a statement	翻譯	翻译
interpreter (n)	one who translates orally from one language into another	譯員	译员
intervention (n)	act or fact of interfering so as to modify	干預	干预
intestinal (adj)	referring to the intestines	腸的	肠的
intestines (n)	the portion of the digestive system extending from the stomach to the anus	腸	肠
intoxicated (adj)	having excess of a toxin, esp. excess alcohol	醉酒的	醉酒的
intramuscular (adj)	within or inside muscle tissue	肌內的	肌内的
intraocular (adj)	within the eye	眼內的	眼内的
intrauterine device (n)	an object that is placed within the uterus to prevent pregnancy	子宮內避孕器	子宫内避孕器
intravenous (adj)	within a vein or veins	靜脈內的	静脉内的
intravenous pyelography (n)	an examination of the kidneys by injecting a liquid visible using x-rays	靜脈腎盂造影術	静脉肾盂造影术
intravenous transfusion (n)	the direct injection of whole blood, plasma, or another solution into the blood stream	靜脈輸液	静脉输液
intubation (n)	insertion of a tube into a body canal or hollow organ, as into the trachea or stomach	插管法	插管法
invasive (adj)	involving puncture or incision of the skin or insertion of an instrument or foreign material into the body	侵入的	侵入的
inverted nipples (n)	nipples that are turned inward	乳頭內翻	乳头内翻
iodine (n)	a grayish-black, corrosive, poisonous element used to clean the skin	碘	碘
iris (n)	the colored, round, membrane of the eye, situated between the cornea and lens	虹膜	虹膜
iritis (n)	inflammation of the iris	虹膜炎	虹膜炎

English/Chinese Medical Glossary - I

iron supplements (n)	an oral medication used to supply the body with additional iron	鐵質補充劑	铁质补充剂
irregular (adj)	not normal; not straight or uniform; having an uneven rate	不正常的，不齊的	不正常的，不齐的
irrigation (n)	washing by a stream of water or other fluid	沖洗法	冲洗法
irritants (n)	something that causes inflammation, soreness, or irritation of a bodily organ or part	刺激劑	刺激剂
irritation (n)	state of over-excitation and extreme sensitivity	刺激，極度敏感	刺激，极度敏感
ischemia (n)	deficiency of blood in a part, due to functional constriction or actual obstruction of a blood vessel	局部缺血	局部缺血
itch (n)	a skin sensation causing a desire to scratch	癢	痒
itch (v)	to feel, have or produce an itch	發癢	发痒

Notes

English/Chinese Medical Glossary - J

jaundice (n)	yellow discoloration of skin, tissues, and body fluids caused by the deposition of bile pigments arising from a variety of conditions that affect the liver	黃疸	黄疸
jaw (n)	the bone holding the lower teeth	頜	颌
jejunum (n)	the middle portion of the small intestine which extends from the duodenum to the ileum	空腸	空肠
jelly (n)	a soft, semi-solid substance used as lubrication and sometimes containing medication or other chemicals, such as spermicidal jelly	凝膠	凝胶
joint (n)	a point of connection between more or less movable parts, between bones, or between segments in the bone	關節	关节
joint socket (n)	the hollow part of a joint that receives the end of a bone	套管接頭	套管接头

Notes

English/Chinese Medical Glossary - K

keratitis (n)	inflammation of the cornea causing poor vision and pain	角膜炎	角膜炎
kidney (n)	either of a pair of structures in the back region of the abdominal cavity, functioning to maintain proper water balance, regulate acid-base concentration, and excrete wastes as urine	腎臟	肾脏
kidney failure (n)	loss of function of one or both kidneys, usually caused by disease or infection	腎衰竭	肾衰竭
kidney stone (n)	a small hard mass that has formed in the kidney and may block the ureter	腎結石	肾结石
kilogram (n)	the fundamental unit of mass in the International System, equaling 2.2 pounds	千克，公斤	千克
knee (n)	the joint or region of the human leg that is between the thigh and calf	膝蓋	膝盖
kneecap (n)	patella; a bone that rests on the knee	膝蓋骨	膝盖骨
knuckle (n)	a joint in the finger, esp. the joint where the finger connects to the hand	指節	指节
kyphosis (n)	hunchback; humpback; excessive curve in the back and spine	脊柱後凸，駝背	脊柱后凸，驼背

Notes

English/Chinese Medical Glossary - L

labor (n) (m)	the physical efforts of childbirth	分娩	分娩
labor and delivery (n)	1. an obstetrical unit, usually associated with prepartum (labor) rooms, a delivery unit (rooms) where child birth occurs and post partum areas where a new mother recovers and begins to care for her child; 2. a term that refers to the physiology of child bearing as in a lecture entitled, "The physiology of normal labor and delivery," or to the active process of bearing a child	陣痛和分娩	阵痛和分娩
labor pains (n)	pain associated with childbirth	陣痛	阵痛
laboratory (n)	a room or building equipped for scientific experiment, research, or the evaluation of blood specimens	實驗室	实验室
laboratory technician (n)	a person trained to work and conduct experiments in a laboratory	化驗員	化验员
laboratory test (n)	any of various tests conducted in a laboratory to assist in the diagnosis of a disease	化驗室檢查	化验室检查
labyrinth (n)	the complex section of passages in the inner ear that senses sound and maintains balance	迷路	迷路
laceration (n)	a torn, ragged, mangled wound	撕裂	撕裂
lacrimal gland (n)	a gland near the eye that secretes tears	淚腺	泪腺
lactation (n)	the act of secreting milk	哺乳	哺乳
lactose intolerance (n)	the inability of the body to digest a specific sugar, lactose; this condition is associated with an upset stomach, diarrhea, and stomach pains	不耐乳糖症	不耐乳糖症
laparoscope (n)	an instrument used to view inside the abdominal cavity	腹腔鏡	腹腔镜

English/Chinese Medical Glossary - L

laparoscopic (adj)	of, or pertaining to a medical procedure of visually examining the abdominal cavity with a slender camera	腹腔鏡檢查	腹腔镜检查
large intestine (n)	the section of the digestive system between the small intestine and anus, consisting of the cecum, colon, rectum, and anal canal	大腸	大肠
laryngitis (n)	inflammation of the larynx, a condition causing dryness and soreness of the throat, hoarseness, and cough	喉炎	喉炎
laryngoscope (n)	a tubular instrument or apparatus used to observe the interior of the larynx	喉鏡	喉镜
larynx (n)	the upper part of the respiratory tract containing the vocal cords	喉	喉
laser surgery, laser photo-coagulation (n)	a surgical procedure using a small laser to destroy tissue or make incisions	鐳射手術	激光手术
latent period (n)	seemingly inactive period, as that between exposure of tissue to an injurious agent and the manifestation of response, or that between a stimulation and the response to the stimulus	潛伏期	潜伏期
laxative (n)	agent that acts to promote release of feces	通瀉劑	通泻剂
lay hands on (v)	the act of resting a person's hand in a particular position or location; a belief that a person has the power to heal through touch	觸碰，療傷聖手	触碰，疗伤圣手
lead poisoning (n)	the pathological effects of ingesting or absorbing lead	鉛中毒	铅中毒
leads (n) (m)	a wire that connects a monitoring device to a patient	引線	引线
leg (n)	a limb or appendage used for movement or support	腿	腿

English/Chinese Medical Glossary - L

lens (n) (m)	a carefully ground and molded piece of glass, plastic, or other transparent material used for changing the size or shape of an image	透鏡	透镜
lens (n) (m)	a transparent part of the eye between the iris and the vitreous used to direct light onto the retina	晶狀體	晶状体
leprosy (n)	an infectious disease usually occurring in the tropics, which can range from being non-contagious to contagious, causing deterioration of the skin; Hansen's disease	痲風	麻风
lesion (n)	a mark on the skin, or abnormal growth (tumor)	瘡口	疮口
lethal (adj)	deadly; fatal	致命的	致命的
lethargy (n)	1. abnormal drowsiness or stupor; 2. a condition of indifference	昏睡	昏睡
leukemia (n)	an acute or chronic disease that involves the blood-forming organs; a form of cancer	白血病	白血病
libido (n)	sexual desire	性欲	性欲
lice (n)	any of numerous small, flatbodied, wingless, biting or sucking insects, usually found in hair	蝨子	虱子
licensed practical nurse (n)	a graduate of a school of practical nursing who has passed the practical nursing state board examination and is licensed to administer care, usually working under direction of a licensed physician or registered nurse	持證執業護士	持证执业护士
life support (n)	hospital equipment that maintains the life of a patient who might not be able to survive independently	生命維持	生命维持

English/Chinese Medical Glossary - L

lifestyle (n)	a way of life or style of living that reflects the attitudes and values of an individual or group	生活方式	生活方式
ligament (n)	a band of fibrous tissue that connects bones or cartilage, serving to support and strengthen joints	韌帶	韧带
limbs (n)	one of the jointed appendages of the human, extending from the trunk	肢	肢
limit (n)	a prescribed maximum or minimum amount, quantity, or number	限度	限度
limp (v)	to walk lamely, esp. with irregularity, as in favoring one leg	跛行	跛行
lip (n)	either of two fleshy, muscular folds that together surround the opening of the mouth	嘴唇	嘴唇
liquids (n)	fluids	液體	液体
little finger (n)	the smallest finger on the hand and most distant from the thumb	小指	小指
little toe (n)	the smallest toe on the foot and most distant from the big toe	小趾	小趾
liver (n)	a large gland that secretes bile, helps in blood formation, and is involved in the metabolism of sugars, fats, proteins, minerals, and vitamins	肝	肝
liver cancer (n)	a tumor in which the cancer starts during adulthood in cells in the liver; also called hepatocellular carcinoma	肝癌	肝癌
living will (n)	a legal document that outlines actions that should be taken if the author is seriously ill and can no longer express wishes regarding his or her death	生前遺囑	生前遗嘱

English/Chinese Medical Glossary - L

loading dose (n)	a quantity higher than the average or maintenance dose, for starting a treatment	負荷劑量（首劑量）	负荷剂量 （首剂量）
lobe (n)	more or less well-defined portion of any organ, especially of the brain, lungs, glands, and ear lobe	葉	叶
local (adj)	restricted to one spot or part	局部的	局部的
local anesthesia (n)	anesthetic which causes loss of feeling only on and around the point where it is applied or injected	局部麻醉	局部麻醉
long term care facility (n)	a health care facility that serves patients with medical conditions requiring nursing and/or medical care on an extended basis	長期治療機構	长期治疗机构
lose consciousness (v)	to become unconscious, without awareness, and not capable of voluntary movement	失去知覺	失去知觉
lose weight (v)	to lower body weight through exercise, dieting, or disease	減肥	减肥
lotion (n)	a medicated liquid for external application	洗液	洗液
low voice (n)	a voice that is not loud; silent	低聲	低声
lower (adj)	below something or someone; below a particular level	較低的	较低的
lower back, lumbar (n)	the region of the back behind the stomach and above the waist	下背，腰部	下背， 腰部
lower jaw (n)	mandible; the movable bone forming the chin and lower portion of the face; it is used in chewing and crushing food	下頜	下颌
lubricant (n)	an oily substance, such as grease, that reduces friction, heat, and wear when applied as a surface coating	潤滑劑	润滑剂
lukewarm (adj)	mildly warm	濕熱的	湿热的
lumbar (adj)	the lower back between the ribs and the pelvis	腰部的	腰部的

English/Chinese Medical Glossary - L

lumbar puncture, spinal tap (n)	the removal of fluid from the spine to assist in diagnosing a disease, such as meningitis	腰椎穿刺，脊椎穿刺	腰椎穿刺，脊椎穿刺
lump (n)	a swelling or small mass	腫塊	肿块
lumpectomy (n)	the removal of a lump	腫瘤切除術	肿瘤切除术
lung (n)	either of two spongy, saclike respiratory organs occupying the chest cavity together with the heart, and functioning to remove carbon dioxide from the blood and provide the body with oxygen	肺	肺
lung cancer (n)	cancer of the lung which is not of the small cell carcinoma (oat cell carcinoma) type; this is generally applied to the various types of bronchogenic carcinomas (those arising from the lining of the bronchi) which include adenocarcinoma, squamous cell carcinoma, and large cell undifferentiated carcinoma	肺癌	肺癌
lung scan (n)	a procedure in which radiation material is injected into the blood to diagnose diseases of the lungs	肺部掃描	肺部扫描
lymph (n)	a clear, transparent, sometimes faintly yellowish liquid that contains white blood cells and some red blood cells and acts to remove bacteria and certain proteins from tissues	淋巴	淋巴
lymph glands (n)	lymph nodes; glands found throughout the body that produce a clear, transparent, sometimes faintly yellowish liquid that contains white blood cells and some red blood cells and acts to remove bacteria and certain proteins from tissues; involved in fighting infection	淋巴結	淋巴结

English/Chinese Medical Glossary - L

lymphadenopathy (n)	enlargement of the lymph nodes	淋巴結病	淋巴结病
lymphatic system (n)	the interconnected system of spaces and vessels between tissues and organs by which lymph is circulated throughout the body	淋巴系統	淋巴系统
lymphoma (n)	a cancerous tumor of lymphoid tissue	淋巴瘤	淋巴瘤

Notes

English/Chinese Medical Glossary - M

magnetic resonance imaging (n)	a diagnostic procedure using magnetic fields (rather than x-ray radiation) to create an image of internal soft tissue, such as muscle, brain, and spinal cord	核磁共振	核磁共振
major depression (n)	a state of depression which includes symptoms of lethargy, sleep disturbance, despondency, morbid thoughts, feelings of worthlessness, and sometimes attempted suicide	嚴重抑鬱症	严重抑郁症
malabsorption (n)	impaired intestinal absorption of nutrients	營養吸收障礙	营养吸收障碍
malaise (n)	a vague feeling of bodily discomfort	不適	不适
malaria (n)	an acute and sometimes chronic disease caused by a microorganism that infects red blood cells, transmitted by the bite of a mosquito	瘧疾	疟疾
malignant (adj)	tending to become progressively worse and to result in death, usually referring to cancer or very serious illness	惡性的	恶性的
malnutrition (n)	inadequate nutrition because of defective digestion or inadequate food intake	營養不良	营养不良
malpractice (n)	improper treatment of a patient by a physician, resulting in damage or injury	療法失當	疗法失当
mammary (n)	the breast	乳房	乳房
mammography, mammogram (n)	1. the practice of taking an x-ray photograph of the breast; 2. an x-ray photograph of the breast	乳房X光攝影術 乳房X光像	乳房照影术, 乳房X光照片
manage (v)	to handle or direct with a degree of skill; to work upon or try to alter for a purpose	管理	管理

English/Chinese Medical Glossary - M

English	Definition	Traditional	Simplified
managed care (n)	a comprehensive approach to the provision of health care that combines clinical services and administrative procedures within an integrated, coordinated system to provide timely access to primary care and other necessary services cost effectively	管理式醫療	管理式医疗
Managed Care Organization (MCO) (n)	health insurance that contracts with health care providers and facilities to deliver services to members at a controlled cost	管理式醫療組織	管理式医疗组织
Managed Health Care Plan (n)	one or more products that integrate financing and management with the delivery of health care services to an enrolled population	管理式健康醫療計劃	管理式健康医疗计划
management (n)	control and oversight	管理	管理
mandible (n)	lower jaw; the movable bone forming the chin and lower portion of the face; it is used in chewing and crushing food	上頜	上颌
mania (n)	a mental disorder characterized by rapidly changing ideas, exaggerated walking stride, increased energy, physical over-activity, and confusion	躁狂	躁狂
manic (adj)	affected with mania	躁狂的	躁狂的
mass (n)	a unified body of matter with no specific shape, sometimes referring to a tumor	塊	块
massage (n)	the systematic therapeutic friction, stroking, and kneading of the body	按摩	按摩
mastectomy (n)	surgical removal of a breast	乳房切除術	乳房切除术
mastitis (n)	inflammation of the mammary gland, or breast	乳腺炎	乳腺炎
masturbation (n)	self-excitation of the genital organs, usually to orgasm, by manual contact or means other than sexual intercourse	手淫	手淫

English/Chinese Medical Glossary - M

maternity ward (n)	a location in a hospital where a woman who is preparing to give birth or just gave birth resides	產科病房	产科病房
measles (n)	an acute, contagious viral disease, usually occurring in childhood and characterized by red spots on the skin	麻疹	麻疹
measure (v)	to determine the dimensions, quantity, or capacity of something	衡量	衡量
Medicaid (Title XIX) (n)	authorized by Title XIX of the Social Security Act, the Medicaid program provides medical benefits for certain low-income persons	醫療補助計劃（《社會安全法案》第十九條）	医疗补助计划（《社会安全法案》第十九条）
medical (adj)	anything having to do with medicine or with the treatment of diseases	醫療的	医疗的
medical alert bracelet (n)	bracelet used for the purpose of identifying the person's medical condition and emergency contact person	醫療警報手鐲	医疗警报手镯
medical assistant (n)	an individual who assists a qualified physician in an office or other clinical setting	醫療助理	医疗助理
Medical Director (n)	a physician responsible for clinical decisions in a health plan or health network	醫療顧問	医疗顾问
medical history (n)	the medical background of a patient, including allergies, past injuries, and diseases	病歷	病历
medical necessity (n)	the determination that an intervention recommended by a treating practitioner is (1) the most appropriate available supply or level of service for the individual in question, considering potential benefits and harms to the individual, and (2) known to be effective in improving health outcomes	醫療必要性	医疗必要性

English/Chinese Medical Glossary - M

medical records (n)	an organized database or file that contains the medical history of one or more patients, contained in a paper chart or on a computer	醫病案	医病案
medical student (n)	a person who is training to be a physician	醫科學生	医科学生
Medicare (Title XVIII) (n)	Title XVIII of the Social Security Act which provides for medical and health services to persons age 65 and older and certain disabled individuals	醫療保險（《社會保障法案》第十八條標題）	医疗保险（《社会保障法案》第十八条标题）
medication (n)	substance given for healing or treatment purposes	醫藥	医药
medicinal (adj)	having healing qualities	醫藥的	医药的
medicine (n)	the science of diagnosing, treating, or preventing disease and other damage to the body or mind	藥物	药物
medicine chest (n)	a storage container for medicine or remedies	藥箱	药箱
meditate (v)	to reflect upon; to ponder	沉思	沉思
meditation (n)	the act or process of meditating	沉思	沉思
melanoma (n)	a tumor of the skin	黑色素瘤	黑色素瘤
melena (n)	the passage of dark (often black) stools stained with blood pigments or with altered blood	黑糞症	黑粪症
member (n)	a person who belongs to an HMO or other health care provider organization; used interchangeably with enrollee and beneficiary	會員	会员
membrane (n)	thin layer of tissue that covers a surface, lines a cavity or divides a space or organ	膈膜	膈膜
memory (n)	the collection of thoughts or images of past events, experiences, knowledge, ideas, and feelings	記憶力	记忆力

English/Chinese Medical Glossary - M

menarche (n)	establishment or beginning of menstrual function in a girl or young woman	初經，月經初潮	初经，月经初潮
menopause (n)	the end of menstruation in the human female, usually in mid life	絕經	绝经
menses (n)	blood and dead cell debris that is discharged from the uterus through the vagina by adult women at approximately monthly intervals between puberty and menopause	月經	月经
menstrual (adj)	of, or pertaining to menstruation	月經的	月经的
menstrual period (n)	the period of time one experiences menstruation each month	月經期	月经期
menstruation (n)	the cyclic, physiologic discharge through the vagina of blood and dead cells from the non-pregnant uterus	月經	月经
mental (adj)	of, or pertaining to the mind; psychic	精神的	精神的
mental health (n)	a section of the medical profession that specializes in the study and treatment of diseases and disorders related to the mind	心理健康	心理健康
mental health professional (n)	a person whose work is related to mental health care	心理健康專家	心理健康专家
mental hospital (n)	a hospital that specializes in treating the mentally ill	精神病院	精神病院
mental illness (n)	any disorder of the mind or psyche	精神病	精神病
mental retardation (n)	mental deficiency; slowed or delayed mental response or activity	精神發育遲緩	精神发育迟缓
mesentery (n)	a membranous fold attaching various organs to the body wall	腸系膜	肠系膜
metabolism (n)	the complex of physical and chemical processes involved in the maintenance of life	新陳代謝	新陈代谢

English/Chinese Medical Glossary - M

English	Definition	Traditional	Simplified
metastasize (v)	to transmit a disease from an original site to one or more sites elsewhere in the body	轉移	转移
metastatic (adj)	of, or pertaining to the transmission of a disease from an original site to one or more sites elsewhere in the body	轉移的	转移的
microorganism (n)	a very small organism, not visible by the human eye without mechanical or electronic magnification	微生物	微生物
microscope (n)	an instrument that uses a combination of lenses to enlarge an image of an object so that it can be seen with the eye	顯微鏡	显微镜
middle ear (n)	the middle section of the ear or tympanic cavity involved in hearing; contains the malleus, incus, and stapes	中耳	中耳
middle finger (n)	the second finger from the thumb	中指	中指
midwife (n)	a person who assists a pregnant woman in childbirth	助產士	助产士
migraine (n)	severe headache, usually affecting only one side of the head, characterized by sharp pain and often accompanied by nausea	偏頭痛	偏头痛
milk (n)	a secretion of a mammary gland that serves as nourishment for the young	乳	乳
mineral (n)	any of various inorganic elements, that are not from an animal or plant, which may be required to live and function properly	無機物，礦物質	无机物，矿物质
mineral supplements (n)	oral medication used to make up for a deficiency in one or more minerals in the body	無機物補充劑	无机物补充剂
miscarriage (n)	a spontaneous, unplanned expulsion of a fetus from the uterus	流產	流产

English/Chinese Medical Glossary - M

misery (n)	a condition or feeling of unhappiness, suffering, or discomfort	痛苦	痛苦
mobility (n)	1. the extent of one's movement; 2. ability to be moved, or to move freely	可動性	可动性
moderation (n)	within reasonable limits, not excessive or extreme	適度	适度
modify (v)	to change somewhat the form or qualities of; to alter partially	調整	调整
moist heat (n)	heat and moisture applied to the skin	濕熱	湿热
moisture (n)	liquid on a surface, giving it a damp feeling or sensation	濕氣	湿气
molar (n)	a tooth with a surface for grinding food, located in the back of the mouth	臼齒	臼齿
mold (n) (m)	a frame or mold around or on which something is formed or shaped	模型	模型
mold (n) (m)	any of various fungous growths	黴	霉
mole, blemish (n)	a small congenital growth on the skin, usually slightly raised and dark, and sometimes hairy	痣	痣
monitor (n) (m)	an instrument used to keep track of an activity, esp. to record the activity of the lungs, brain, or heart	監視器	监视器
mononucleosis (n)	a temporary illness associated with fatigue and abnormal white blood cells in the blood; also called mono	單核細胞增多	单核细胞增多
mood swing (n)	shift in emotional state, such as happy then sad	情緒波動	情绪波动
morbidity (n)	1. a diseased condition or state; 2. the incidence of a disease or of all diseases in a population	①病態；②發病率	①病态；②发病率

English/Chinese Medical Glossary - M

morning sickness (n)	vomiting and nausea that affects some women during the first few weeks of pregnancy	晨暈	晨晕
mortuary (n)	a place, esp. a funeral home, where dead bodies are kept prior to burial or cremation	停屍室	停尸室
mouth (n)	the body opening through which a human takes in food	嘴	嘴
mouthwash (n)	a flavored liquid for cleaning the mouth and making one's breath smell better	漱口劑	漱口剂
mucous membrane (n)	the moist membrane lining all bodily channels that communicate with the air, such as the respiratory and digestive tracts, the glands of which secrete mucus	粘膜	粘膜
mucus (n)	the free slime of the mucous membranes, composed of secretion of the glands, along with various inorganic salts	粘液	粘液
multidose (n)	occurring in, or using more than one dose	多次劑量	多次剂量
multiparous (adj)	having had one or more previous successful pregnancies	多胎產的	多胎产的
multiple sclerosis (n)	a degenerative disease of the central nervous system resulting in weakness and a variety of neurological symptoms	多發性硬化	多发性硬化
mumps (n)	an acute, inflammatory, contagious disease of the glands that produce saliva	流行性腮腺炎	流行性腮腺炎
muscle (n)	a tissue in the body comprised of fibers which can tighten and relax to produce movement	肌肉	肌肉
muscle relaxant (n)	an agent that specifically aids in reducing muscle tension	肌肉鬆弛劑	肌肉松弛剂
muscular (adj)	of, or pertaining to muscle	肌肉的	肌肉的

English/Chinese Medical Glossary - M

muscular system (n)	the organization and action of muscles in the body that control movement, aid digestion, and help blood circulation	肌系統	肌系统
mute (adj)	unable to speak	啞的	哑的
mycosis (n)	any disease caused by a fungus	黴菌病	霉菌病
myeloma (n)	a tumor composed of cells of the type normally found in the bone marrow	骨髓瘤	骨髓瘤
myocardial infarction (n)	heart attack	心肌梗塞	心肌梗塞
myopia (n)	a condition in which the eye does not focus properly on distant objects without the aid of glasses; nearsightedness	近視	近视

Notes

English/Chinese Medical Glossary - N

nail (finger or toe) (n) (m)	the hard, horn-like substance that naturally grows at the end of a finger or toe	（手或腳）指甲	（手或脚）指甲
narcotic (n)	any natural or synthetic drug that has morphine-like actions; a painkiller	麻醉劑	麻醉剂
nasal (adj)	of, or pertaining to the nose	鼻的	鼻的
nasal congestion (n)	a condition where excess mucus in the nose makes breathing difficult	鼻充血	鼻充血
nasal irrigation (n)	a procedure where the nasal canal is cleaned with a liquid to treat disease or an infection	鼻沖洗	鼻冲洗
nasal polyp (n)	a growth found in the tissue of the nose	鼻息肉	鼻息肉
nausea (n)	an unpleasant sensation often including vomiting and upset stomach	噁心	恶心
nauseated (adj)	affected with nausea, the state of having an unpleasant sensation often including vomiting and upset stomach	噁心	恶心
nauseous (adj)	of, or pertaining to the feelings of nausea	噁心的	恶心的
navel (n)	the mark left on the abdomen where the umbilical cord was attached; belly button	肚臍	肚脐
nearsighted (adj)	unable to see distant objects clearly	近視的	近视的
neck (n)	the part of the body joining the head to the trunk	頸	颈
needle aspiration biopsy (n)	a procedure involving the removal of fluid from any tissue of the body with a needle or aspiration device, used in diagnosis of a disease	針吸活檢	针吸活检
needle, syringe (n)	a medical instrument used to inject fluids into the body or draw them from it	注射針	注射针
negative (adj)	not affirming the presence of the organism or condition in question; lacking the quality of being positive	陰性的	阴性的

English/Chinese Medical Glossary - N

neonatal (adj)	of, or pertaining to the first four weeks after birth	新生期的	新生期的
neonatologist (n)	a physician who specializes in the care and treatment of infants within the first 28 days of birth	新生兒學專家	新生儿学专家
neoplasm (n)	an abnormal new growth of tissue; tumor	腫瘤	肿瘤
nephritis (n)	inflammation of the kidney	腎炎	肾炎
nephrologist (n)	a physician whose specializes in the study of the kidneys	腎病學家	肾病学家
nephrology (n)	the medical study of the structure and function of the kidneys	腎病學	肾病学
nerve (n)	any of the bundles of fibers capable of sending both sensory and motor signals from one part of the body to another; a fiber that enables movement and feeling	神經	神经
nervous (adj)	of, or pertaining to a nerve or the activity of a nerve	神經的	神经的
nervous system (n)	the network of nerves, extending throughout the body, that control movement, feeling, etc.	神經系統	神经系统
nervousness (n)	excessive excitability and irritability, with mental and physical unrest	神經過敏	神经过敏
neurologist (n)	a person who studies the medical science of the nervous system and its disorders	神經病學家	神经病学家
neurology (n)	the medical science of the nervous system and its disorders	神經病學	神经病学
neuropathy (n)	any and all disease or malfunction of the nerves	神經病	神经病
neurosis (n)	any of various functional disorders of the mind or emotions without obvious damage or change to the brain	神經質	神经质
neurosurgery (n)	surgery of any part of the nervous system	神經外科學	神经外科学

English/Chinese Medical Glossary - N

neurotic (adj)	a person with excessive worries	神經機能病的	神经机能病的
neurotoxic (adj)	poisonous or destructive to nerve tissue	神經中毒的	神经中毒的
neutral (adj) (m)	1. not allied with, supporting, or favoring either side; indifferent; 2. not acidic or basic	中性的	中性的
neutralization (n)	an act or process of neutralizing	中合作用	中合作用
next of kin (n)	the person most closely related to a person	最近的血親	最近的血亲
nicotine patch (n)	a patch worn on the skin that helps reduce the addiction to tobacco	尼古丁貼片	尼古丁贴片
nicotine replacement aids (n)	a nicotine-replacement aid placed in a smoker's mouth to help reduce the habit of using tobacco; the nicotine in the gum passes through the mucous membranes of the mouth	尼古丁替代療法	尼古丁替代疗法
night blindness (n)	the inability to see in the dark	夜盲症	夜盲症
nipple (n)	the small projection near the center of the mammary gland or breast containing outlets of milk ducts	乳頭	乳头
nitroglycerin (n)	medication used to open blood vessels	硝酸甘油	硝酸甘油
nocturnal (adj)	occurring at, or active at night	夜間的	夜间的
nodule (n)	a small node, as of body tissue; a localized swelling	小結	小结
non-contagious (adj)	not communicable	非傳染疾病	非传染疾病
non-medical home equipment (n)	assistive devices, appliances & supplies which are necessary to assure the client's health, safety and independence	非醫療居家設備	非医疗居家设备
non-medical transportation (n)	transportation of members by passenger car, taxicabs, or other forms of public or private conveyances	非醫療交通	非医疗交通

English/Chinese Medical Glossary - N

English	Definition	繁體	简体
Non-Physician Medical Practitioners (Mid-Level Practitioner) (n)	a nurse practitioner, nurse midwife, or physician assistant allowed to provide primary care under physician supervision	非醫師的執業治療師（中級治療師）	非医师的执业 治疗师（中级治疗师）
nonspecific (adj)	not due to any single known cause	非特異性的	非特异性的
non-stress test (n)	a test to evaluate fetal well-being by evaluating fetal heart rate response to fetal movement	非應激試驗	非应激试验
normal (adj)	usual, standard, or typical	正常的	正常的
nose (n)	the structure of the face or forward part of the head that contains the organs of smell and forms the beginning of the respiratory tract	鼻	鼻
nose drops (n)	a medication administered in drops into the nose	滴鼻劑	滴鼻剂
nose spray (n)	a medication administered as a mist into the nose	鼻噴劑	鼻喷剂
nosebleed (n)	bleeding from the nose	鼻出血	鼻出血
nostril (n)	either of the external openings of the nose	鼻孔	鼻孔
nothing by mouth (n)	an instruction by a physician to not eat or drink, usually for a number of hours prior to surgery, or in preparation for a diagnostic test	禁食	禁食
numb (adj)	lacking the power to feel pain or touch	麻木的	麻木的
nurse (v)	to feed with milk from the breast; to suckle	護理	护理
nurse practitioner (n)	a registered nurse who can work independently of a physician and provide all levels of care to patients, including treatments and prescriptions	護理師	护理师
nursing home (n)	a private hospital for the care of the aged or chronically ill	療養院	疗养院
nutrient (n)	an important substance for function of the body; food, or a component of food	營養素	营养素

English/Chinese Medical Glossary - N

nutrition (n)	the process of nourishing or being nourished, esp. the process by which humans digest food and use it for growth and for replacement of tissue	營養物	营养物
nutritional supplement (n)	a product intended for ingestion to add to or to complete a diet and that contains one or more of the following dietary ingredients: a vitamin, mineral, amino acid, herb or other botanical	營養補劑	营养补剂
nutritionist (n)	a person who specializes in the study of nutrition	營養學家	营养学家

Notes

English/Chinese Medical Glossary - O

obese (adj)	extremely fat; overweight	肥胖的	肥胖的
obesity (n)	an increase in body weight; an excessive accumulation of fat in the body	肥胖	肥胖
observation (n)	the act of watching attentively	觀察	观察
obstetric nurse (n)	a nurse specialized in caring for pregnant women	助產師	助产士
obstetrician (n)	a physician specializing in obstetrics	產科醫師	产科医师
obstetrics (n)	branch of medicine that deals with pregnancy, childbirth, and the post-partum period	產科學	产科学
obstruction (n)	act of blocking or clogging	梗阻	梗阻
occipital (adj)	of, or pertaining to the back of the head, esp. the posterior part of the skull	枕骨的	枕骨的
occult (adj)	hidden from view; concealed from observation; difficult to understand	隱的	隐的
occult blood (n)	blood that cannot be seen, but is identified by using special techniques, usually referring to blood in the stool	大便潛血	大便潜血
occupational disease (n)	a disease caused by work-related activities	職業病	职业病
ocular (adj)	of, or pertaining to the eye; seen by the eye	眼的	眼的
oculist (n)	a physician who treats disease of the eyes; ophthalmologist	眼科醫師	眼科医师
oil (n)	any of numerous mineral, vegetable, and man-made substances and animal and vegetable fats that are generally slippery, inflammable, and liquid at room temperatures	油	油
ointment (n)	a medication applied to the skin	軟膏	软膏
on an empty stomach (prep)	describing a physical state of not having eaten for an extended period, thereby having digested all the food in the stomach	空腹時	空腹时

English/Chinese Medical Glossary - O

oncologist (n)	a physician who specializes in the study of cancer	腫瘤學家	肿瘤学家
onset (n)	the beginning, esp. of an illness	起始	起始
ooze (v)	to flow or leak out slowly, as through small openings	滲出	渗出
operate (v) (m)	to perform surgery	動手術	动手术
operating room (n)	a section of a hospital where surgical procedures are performed	手術室	手术室
operation (n) (m)	a procedure for repairing or relieving an injury, ailment, or dysfunction in a living body, esp. performed with instruments; surgery	手術	手术
ophthalmic (adj)	pertaining to the eye	眼睛的	眼睛的
ophthalmologic (adj)	of, or pertaining to the branch of medicine dealing with the eye	眼科學的	眼科学的
ophthalmologist (n)	a physician who specializes in the anatomy, functions, pathology, and treatment of the eye	眼科醫師	眼科医师
ophthalmology (n)	the branch of medicine dealing with the eye	眼科學	眼科学
opiate (n)	a remedy containing or derived from opium; also any drug that induces sleep or relieves pain	鴉片製劑	鸦片制剂
optic (adj)	of, or pertaining to the eye	視覺的	视觉的
optic nerve (n)	the nerve that delivers signals from the eye to the brain	視神經	视神经
optimal (adj)	the best; the most favorable	最適的	最适的
optometrist (n)	a person whose profession is examining, measuring, and treating certain visual defects by means of corrective lenses or other methods that do not require a physician's license	驗光師	验光师

English/Chinese Medical Glossary - O

optometry (n)	the profession of examining, measuring, and treating certain visual defects by means of corrective lenses or other methods that do not require license as a physician	視力測定法	视力测定法
oral (adj)	1. pertaining to the mouth (adj); 2. taken through or applied in the mouth (adv)	口內的	口的
oral cavity (n)	the mouth	口腔	口腔
oral surgery (n)	surgery specific to the mouth	口腔外科	口腔外科
organ (n)	a differentiated part of the human, adapted for a specific function, such as the heart or lungs	器官	器官
organ donor (n)	a person who gives an organ to another patient	器官捐獻者	器官捐献者
orthodontist (n)	a dentist who specializes in the practice of correcting abnormally aligned or positioned teeth	矯形齒科醫師	矫形齿科医师
orthopedics (n)	the study of the musculoskeletal system	骨科矯形學	骨科矫形学
orthopedist (n)	a physician who specializes in the surgical or manipulative treatment of disorders of the skeletal system and associated motor organs	骨科矯形醫師	骨科矫形医师
ossicle (n)	a small ear bone	小骨	小骨
osteoarthritis (n)	degenerative joint disease	骨關節炎	骨关节炎
osteoporosis (n)	reduction in the amount of bone mass, leading to fractures after minimal trauma	骨質疏鬆症	骨质疏松症
osteotomy (n)	the surgical cutting of a bone	骨切開術	骨切开术
otitis (n)	inflammation of the ear, which may be marked by pain, fever, abnormalities of hearing, etc.	耳炎	耳炎
otoscope (n)	a device used to examine the ear	耳鏡	耳镜
outer ear (n)	the portion of the ear that consists of the auricle and ear canal	外耳	外耳

English/Chinese Medical Glossary - O

outpatient (n)	a patient who receives treatment at a hospital or clinic without being hospitalized	門診病人	门诊病人
ovarian (adj)	pertaining to an ovary or ovaries	卵巢的	卵巢的
ovarian cyst (n)	a cyst that has grown on or originated from an ovary	卵巢囊腫	卵巢囊肿
ovary (n)	one of a pair of female reproductive glands located on both sides of the uterus	卵巢	卵巢
over the counter (drugs) (prep/n)	medication that can be purchased without a prescription	非處方藥	非处方药
overactive thyroid (n)	hyperthyroidism; excessive production of thyroid hormone	甲狀腺亢進	甲狀腺亢进
overdosage (n)	administration of an excessive dose; condition resulting from an excessive dose	過劑量	过剂量
overdose (n)	an excessive dose	過度劑量	过度剂量
ovulation (n)	the period during a woman's monthly cycle where a mature egg is released, making her very susceptible to pregnancy	排卵	排卵
oxygen (n)	a colorless, odorless, tasteless gaseous element essential for respiration and essential for human life	氧氣	氧气
oxygenation (n)	process of supplying, treating, or mixing with oxygen	氧合	氧合

Notes

English/Chinese Medical Glossary - O

English/Chinese Medical Glossary - P

pacemaker (n)	a device which influences the rate of the heart	起搏器	起搏器
pain (n)	an unpleasant sensation, occurring in varying degrees of severity as a consequence of injury, disease, or emotional disorder	疼痛	疼痛
pain constant (n)	pain that continues without subsiding	疼痛持續	疼痛持续
pain dull (n)	pain that is not intensely or keenly felt	隱痛	隐痛
pain killer (n)	something, such as a drug, that relieves pain	止痛藥	止痛药
pain on and off (n)	pain that is felt and then is not felt	陣痛	阵痛
pain radiating (n)	discomfort that originates from a central location and spreads outward, esp. down the arm and shoulder	疼痛擴散	疼痛扩散
pain sharp (n)	pain that is harsh or biting	銳痛	锐痛
pain shooting (n)	a sudden intense feeling of pain or discomfort	刺痛	刺痛
pain throbbing (n)	pain that vibrates, pulsates, or has a rhythm	抽痛	抽痛
painful (adj)	causing pain; hurtful	疼痛的	疼痛的
palate (n)	the roof of the mouth consisting of a bony front, the hard palate, backed by the fleshy soft palate	顎	颚
pale (adj)	whitish, referring to skin color	蒼白的	苍白的
palliative (adj)	of, or pertaining to medical treatment affording relief, but no cure	姑息的	姑息的
pallor (n)	extreme or unnatural paleness	蒼白	苍白
palm (n)	the inner surface of the hand, extending from the wrist to the base of the fingers	手掌	手掌
palpitation (n)	a rapid or irregular heart beat; the act of shaking, quivering, or fluttering	心悸	心悸

English/Chinese Medical Glossary - P

pamphlet (n)	a piece of folded paper printed with information about a procedure, program, disease, or health issue	小冊子	小册子
pancreas (n)	a long, soft, irregularly shaped gland lying behind the stomach that helps with digestion and metabolism	胰臟	胰脏
pancreatitis (n)	acute or chronic inflammation of the pancreas	胰腺炎	胰腺炎
pap smear, pap test (n)	a procedure in which cells are collected from the cervix and examined for cancer	子宮頸抹片，子宮頸抹片檢查	子宫颈抹片，子宫颈抹片检查
paralysis (n)	loss or impairment of motor function	癱瘓	瘫痪
paramedic (n)	a person who is trained to supply emergency medical treatment or to assist medical professionals	急救人員	急救人员
paranoia (n)	a very unstable mental condition in which the person has a feeling of being in danger, chased, or threatened	偏執狂	偏执狂
paraplegia (n)	paralysis of the legs and lower part of the body	截癱	截瘫
parasite (n)	an organism that grows, feeds, and lives on or in another organism, usually causing harm to the other organism	寄生物	寄生物
parasitic (adj)	of, or pertaining to, or caused by a parasite	寄生的	寄生的
parathyroid (n)	one of four glands situated beside the thyroid gland that are involved in hormone secretion	副甲狀腺	副甲状腺
parenting (v)	caring for children	養育	养育
paresthesia (n)	abnormal or impaired skin sensation, such as burning, prickling, itching, or tingling	感覺異常	感觉异常
parietal (adj)	1. of, or pertaining to the walls of a cavity; 2. of, or pertaining to a specific portion of the skull	壁的	壁的

English/Chinese Medical Glossary - P

Parkinson's Disease (n)	a progressive nervous disease of older people, characterized by involuntary movements, partial facial paralysis, difficulty walking, and general weakness	帕金森氏病	帕金森氏病
partner (n)	one associated with another, especially in an action	夥伴，配偶體	伙伴，配偶体
pass out (v)	to become unconscious, without awareness, and not capable of voluntary movement	昏倒	昏倒
pasta (n)	a food, such as spaghetti, made from water and flour and formed into different shapes then cooked in boiling water; it is high in carbohydrates	〔義大利〕麵	（義大利）麵
patella (n)	kneecap; a flat, triangular bone located at the front of the knee joint	膝蓋骨	膝盖骨
pathogen (n)	any disease-producing microorganism	病原體	病原体
pathogenic (adj)	capable of causing a disease	致病的	致病的
pathologic (adj)	pathological; of, or pertaining to pathology; pertaining to or caused by disease	病理的	病理的
pathologist (n)	a person who specializes in the study of pathology	病理學家	病理学家
pathology (n)	the scientific study of the nature of disease, its causes, processes, development, and consequences	病理學	病理学
patient (n)	person receiving medical treatment	病人	病人

English/Chinese Medical Glossary - P

English	Definition	Traditional	Simplified
patient advocate (n)	a person who argues for a patient, who supports a patient in gaining equal access to health care (this is different than an interpreter taking on the advocate role, which is an action an interpreter takes on behalf of the patient outside the bounds of an interpreted interview)	維權者	维权者
peak-flow meter (n)	a hand-held device that measures air flow (how fast air is blown out of the lungs); patients can use peak-flow meters to measure their own air flow regularly	最大呼氣流量計	最大呼气流量计
pediatric nurse practitioner (n)	a registered nurse with advanced training who provides primary health care to children	兒科護理專家	儿科护理专家
pediatrician (n)	a physician who specializes in the care and medical treatment of children	兒科醫師	儿科医师
pediatrics (n)	care and medical treatment of children	小兒科	小儿科
pelvic (adj)	of, or pertaining to the pelvis	骨盆的	骨盆的
pelvic inflammatory disease (n)	infection of the uterus and adjacent pelvic structures	骨盆腔發炎	骨盆腔发炎
pelvis (n)	a basin-shaped skeletal structure that rests on the bones of the lower limbs and supports the spinal column	盆骨	盆骨
penetration (n)	act of piercing or entering deeply	穿透術	穿透术
penis (n)	male organ of sexual intercourse and of urinary excretion	陰莖	阴茎
peptic (adj)	of, or pertaining to, or assisting digestion	消化的	消化的

English/Chinese Medical Glossary - P

peptic ulcer disease (n)	a hole in the lining of the stomach, duodenum, or esophagus; a peptic ulcer occurs when the lining of these organs is corroded by the acidic digestive juices that are secreted by the stomach cells	消化性潰瘍病	消化性溃疡病
percutaneous (adj)	performed through the skin, as injection	經皮的	经皮的
perforation (n)	act of boring or piercing through a part	穿孔	穿孔
perinatal (adj)	pertaining to or occurring in the period shortly before and after birth	圍產期的	围产期的
perineum (n)	the portion of the body in the pelvis occupied by the bladder, uterus, ovaries, rectum, etc., bounded in front by the pubic arch, in back by the tailbone, and to the sides by the hipbone	會陰	会阴
period (menstrual) (n) (m)	an instance or occurrence of menstruation	經期	经期
period (related to time) (n) (m)	an interval of time characterized by the occurrence of certain conditions or events	週期	周期
periodontal disease (n)	a disease of the tissue and structures surrounding and supporting the teeth	牙周病	牙周病
periosteum (n)	the fibrous membrane covering bone that supports blood vessels and the attachment of ligaments, tendons, and muscles	骨膜	骨膜
persistent (adj)	continuing to exist in spite of interference or treatment; tending to recur	持續的	持续的
personal care (adj)	provides assistance to maintain bodily hygiene, personal safety, and activities of daily living	個人護理	个人护理
perspiration (n)	sweating; the functional secretion of sweat	出汗	出汗

English/Chinese Medical Glossary - P

perspire (v)	to excrete sweat or perspiration through the pores of the skin	出汗	出汗
pertussis (n)	an acute, highly contagious infection of the respiratory tract, causing a harsh cough; most frequently affecting young children	百日咳	百日咳
pessary (n)	instrument placed in the vagina to support the uterus or rectum or as a device to prevent pregnancy	子宮托	子宫托
phallic (adj)	pertaining to the penis	陰莖的	阴茎的
pharmacist (n)	a person trained in pharmacy; druggist	藥劑師	药剂师
pharmacy (n)	a place where medicines are prepared and sold	藥劑學	药剂学
pharynx (n)	the section of throat that allows for the passage of air and the passage of food	咽	咽
phlebitis (n)	inflammation of a vein	靜脈炎	静脉炎
phlegm (n)	stringy, thick mucus	粘痰	粘痰
phobia (n)	persistent, irrational, intense fear of a specific object, activity, or situation	恐怖症	恐怖症
photophobia (n)	abnormal visual intolerance of light	畏光	畏光
physical (adj)	pertaining to the body, to material things, or to physics	體力的	体力的
physical exam (n)	a general examination of the body for any diseases, disorders, or pathogenic conditions	體檢	体检
physical therapist (n)	a person trained to treat disease and injury by mechanical means, such as exercise, heat, light, and massage	理療師	理疗师
physical therapy (n)	the treatment of disease and injury by mechanical means, such as exercise, heat, light, and massage	物理治療法	物理治疗法

English/Chinese Medical Glossary - P

physician (n)	doctor; a person trained in the healing arts and licensed to practice	醫師	医师
physician's assistant (n)	a person trained to assist a physician in procedures and examination of patients	助理醫師	助理医师
pigment (n)	a substance used as coloring	色素	色素
pigmentation (n)	coloration of tissues by pigment	色素沉著	色素沉着
piles (n)	hemorrhoids	痔 (n)	痔 (n)
pill (n)	a small pellet or tablet of medicine, often coated, taken by swallowing whole or chewing	藥片	药片
pillow (n)	a soft stuffed cloth cushion used to rest the head, esp. during sleep	枕頭	枕头
pimple (n)	a small swelling of the skin, sometimes containing pus	膿皰	脓疱
pituitary gland (n)	a small, oval endocrine gland attached to the base of the brain that controls growth, maturation, and metabolism	腦下垂體	脑下垂体
placebo (n)	a medication or treatment known to have no effect, often used for comparison in an experiment	安慰劑	安慰剂
placenta (n)	an organ located in the uterus that joins a mother to her unborn baby and through which it receives nourishment	胎盤	胎盘
plague (n)	a highly infectious, usually fatal, epidemic disease	鼠疫	鼠疫
plasma (n)	the liquid part of blood	血漿	血浆
plastic surgery (n)	surgery to remodel, repair, or restore injured or defective body parts, esp. by transfer of tissue	整形手術	整形手术
platelets (n)	a disk, smaller than a red blood cell, found in the blood, which helps prevent bleeding	血小板	血小板

English/Chinese Medical Glossary - P

pleura (n)	either of two sacs, each of which lines one side of the chest cavity and holds the lungs	胸膜	胸膜
pleural cavity (n)	the space within the pleura where the lungs are located	胸膜腔	胸膜腔
pleural effusion (n)	the escape of fluid from the blood vessels in the pleural cavity	胸膜腔滲液	胸膜腔渗液
pleural rub (n)	friction of one surface moving over another causing inflammation of the pleural cavity	胸膜摩擦音	胸膜摩擦音
pleurisy (n)	inflammation of the pleural cavity	胸膜炎	胸膜炎
plugged ear (n)	a condition in which there is a clot, usually of ear wax, in the ear canal, causing difficulties in hearing	耳塞	耳塞
pneumococcal pneumonia (n)	lung infection caused by Streptococcus pneumoniae	肺炎球菌性肺炎	肺炎球菌性肺炎
pneumonia (n)	inflammation of the lungs caused by virus, bacteria, and physical and chemical agents	肺炎	肺炎
pneumothorax (n)	accumulation of air or gas in the pleural cavity, occurring as a result of disease or injury	氣胸	气胸
podiatrist (n)	a person whose profession is the study and treatment of foot problems	腳病醫師	脚病医师
poison (n)	a substance that causes injury, illness, or death, esp. by chemical means	毒藥	毒药
policy (n)	a plan or course of action; guiding principle or procedure considered to be expedient, prudent, or advantageous	保險計劃	保险计划
polio (n)	poliomyelitis; an acute viral disease, occurring sporadically and in epidemics, which causes paralysis	小兒麻痺症	小儿麻痹症

English/Chinese Medical Glossary - P

pollen (n)	small, light, dry protein particles from trees, grasses, flowers, and weeds that may be spread by the wind; pollen is a potent stimulator of allergic responses	花粉	花粉
pollutant (n)	something that pollutes, esp. a waste material that contaminates air, soil, or water	污染物	污染物
pollute (v)	to make unfit for or harmful to humans, animals and plants, esp. by the addition of waste matter or harmful chemicals	污染	污染
pollution (n)	the act or process of polluting or the state of being polluted; the contamination of the body by the exposure to harmful substances	污染	污染
polyp (n)	a growth protruding from the mucous lining of an organ such as the nose	息肉	息肉
pores (n)	a very small opening in the skin	毛孔	毛孔
positive (adj)	indicating a presence of a particular disease, condition, or organism	陽性的	阳性的
post nasal drip (n)	the chronic secretion of mucus from the posterior nasal cavities, resulting in soreness and congestion of the throat	鼻液倒流	鼻液倒流
posterior (adj)	situated in back of, or in the back part of, or affecting the back or dorsal surface of the body	後的	后的
postmenopausal (adj)	occurring after menopause	經絕後的	经绝后的
postnatal (adj)	occurring after birth, with reference to the newborn	出生後的	出生后的
postoperative (adj)	occurring after a surgical operation	手術後的	手术后的
post-partum (adj)	of, or occurring in the period shortly after childbirth	產後的	产后的

English/Chinese Medical Glossary - P

post-traumatic (adj)	occurring as a result of or after injury	外傷後的	外伤后的
posture (n)	a position or attitude of the body or of bodily parts	姿勢	姿势
pound (n)	a unit of weight equal to 16 ounces	磅	磅
power of attorney (n)	a legal instrument authorizing one to act as another's attorney or agent	委託書，授權書	委托书
preclinical (adj)	before a disease becomes recognizable to a doctor	臨床前的	临床前的
preeclampsia (n)	development of high blood pressure due to pregnancy or the influence of a recent pregnancy	子癇前期	子痫前期
pregnancy (n)	the condition of being pregnant	懷孕	怀孕
pregnancy test (n)	a procedure used to determine if someone is pregnant	驗孕	验孕
pregnant (adj)	carrying a developing baby within the uterus	懷孕的	怀孕的
preload (n)	the load of blood waiting to get into the heart	預負荷	预负荷
premature (adj)	occurring before the proper time, esp. a premature infant	早產兒	早产儿
pre-menstrual (adj)	occurring before menstruation	經前的	经前的
prenatal (adj)	existing or occurring before birth, with reference to the baby	產前的	产前的
prenatal care (n)	medical care given to the mother prior to birth	產前護理	产前护理
pre-operative (adj)	preceding an operation	手術前	手术前
presbyopia (n)	the inability of the eye to focus sharply on nearby objects, usually occurring with advancing age	老視	老视
prescribe (v)	to order or recommend the use of a drug or treatment	開處方	开处方
prescription (n)	a written direction for the preparation and administration of a remedy	處方藥	处方药

English/Chinese Medical Glossary - P

pressure (n)	the act of applying a continuous force on something	壓力	压力
pressure sore (n)	bed sore	褥瘡	褥疮
preteen (n)	child of age group 10 to 12 years old	青春期	青春期
prevent (v)	to keep from happening	預防	预防
preventative (adj)	designed or used to prevent or hinder; thwarting or warding off illness or disease	預防性的	预防性的
preventive care services (n)	services provided to prevent illness; there are three levels of preventive care: primary, such as immunizations, aimed at preventing disease; secondary, such as disease screening programs, aimed at early detection of disease; and tertiary, such as physical therapy, aimed at restoring function after the disease has occurred	預防性護理服務	预防性护理服务
prick (v)	to puncture or poke lightly	扎	扎
primary care physician (PCP) (n)	a physician who focuses his/her practice of medicine on general practice or who is a board certified or board eligible internist, pediatrician, obstetrician/gynecologist, or family practitioner; this physician is responsible for supervising, coordinating, and providing initial and primary care	初級醫療醫生 (PCP) (私人醫生)	初级医疗医生 (PCP) (私人医生)
primary care provider (n)	a person or other health care provider responsible for supervising, coordinating, and providing initial and primary care to patients; this provider is responsible for initiating referrals and maintaining the continuity of patient care	初級醫療提供者	初级医疗提供者

English/Chinese Medical Glossary - P

primary care services (n)	a physician or other health care provider who does not specialize in a particular area but treats a variety of medical problems, usually serving a family	初級醫療服務	初级医疗服务
primary vaccination (n)	first or principal vaccination	初次接種	初次接种
prior authorization review (n)	the process of obtaining prior approval from one's health insurance provider as to the appropriateness of a service or medication; prior authorization does not guarantee insurance coverage	事先授權審查	事先授权审查
procreation (n)	entire process of bringing a new individual into the world	生殖	生殖
prognosis (n)	a forecast as to the probable outcome of an illness or injury; the prospect as to recovery from a disease as indicated by the nature and symptons of the case	預後	预后
program (n)	a plan or system under which action may be taken toward a goal	計劃	计划
progressive (adj)	advancing; going forward; increasing in scope or severity	進行性的	进行性的
prolapse (n)	the falling down, or sinking of an organ or part, such as a prolapse of the uterus	下垂	下垂
proliferation (n)	reproduction or multiplication of similar forms	增生	增生
prophylaxis (n)	prevention of disease; preventive treatment	預防	预防
prostate gland (n)	a gland in males composed of muscular and glandular tissue that surrounds the urethra at the bladder	前列腺	前列腺
prosthesis (n)	an artificial replacement of a missing part of the body, esp. an arm or leg	修復術；假體	修复术；假体

English/Chinese Medical Glossary - P

protective supervision (n)	insures provision of 24 hour supervision to persons in their homes who are very frail or otherwise may suffer a medical emergency, to prevent immediate placement in an acute care hospital, skilled nursing facility, or other 24 –hour care facility	保護性監管	保护性监管
protein (n) (m)	an essential nutrient for growth and survival of the human body	蛋白質	蛋白质
provider (of health care) (n)	a physician, nurse, technician, teacher, hospital, insurance company, health maintenance organization, voluntary agency, or other person or institution engaged in furnishing some type of care to individuals	（健康護理）提供人員	（健康护理）提供人員
pruritus (n)	severe itching, usually of undamaged skin	瘙癢	瘙痒
psoriasis (n)	a chronic, non-contagious skin disease characterized by inflammation and white, scaly patches	牛皮癬	牛皮癣
psychiatrist (n)	a physician who specializes in the study, diagnosis, treatment, and prevention of mental illness	精神病學家	精神病学家
psychologist (n)	a non-physician who specializes in the study of mental processes and behavior	心理學家	心理学家
psychology (n)	the science of mental processes and behavior	心理學	心理学
puberty (n)	the stage of life when an individual becomes capable of sexual reproduction	青春期	青春期
pubic bone (n)	a bone found in the pelvis below the abdomen	恥骨	耻骨
pubic hair (n)	the hair growing around the external genitals	陰毛	阴毛
pubis (n)	the area over the pubic bone, below the abdomen	恥骨	耻骨

English/Chinese Medical Glossary - P

pulmonary abscess (n)	a pus-containing infection in the lung	肺膿腫	肺脓肿
pulmonary angiography (n)	a procedure that examines the blood vessels in the lungs by injecting a substance into the blood vessel and taking an x-ray image	肺動脈造影術	肺动脉造影术
pulmonary artery (n)	an artery that supplies blood to the lungs	肺動脈	肺动脉
pulmonary edema (n)	the presence of excess fluid in the lungs	肺水腫	肺水肿
pulmonary embolism (n)	the obstruction of a blood vessel in a lung	肺栓塞	肺栓塞
pulmonary function tests (n)	one of a number of tests used to determine the ability of the lungs to exchange oxygen and carbon dioxide	肺功能檢查	肺功能检查
pulmonary infarction (n)	a condition where blood cannot be delivered to the lungs; it is usually caused by a blood clot	肺梗塞	肺梗塞
pulmonologist (n)	a physician who specializes in the treatment and study of lung diseases	肺臟學家	肺脏学家
pulse (n)	the throbbing of arteries produced by the regular contractions of the heart	脈搏	脉搏
pump the stomach (v)	a medical procedure used to remove all contents of the stomach in an effort to remove toxic substances	洗胃	洗胃
pupil (of eye) (n) (m)	the apparently black circular area in the center of the eye	（眼睛）瞳孔	（眼睛）瞳孔
purified protein derivative (n)	a test administered by injection to determine if a patient has tuberculosis	純化蛋白衍生物	纯化蛋白衍生物
purulent (adj)	containing or secreting pus	膿性的	脓性的
pus (n)	a yellowish-white fluid, consisting mainly of white blood cells and cellular debris, that forms in infected tissue	膿	脓

English/Chinese Medical Glossary - P

push (v)	to exert force against an object to move it away; to move an object by exerting force against it; to thrust; to shove; to bear hard upon; to press	擠出	挤出
pustule (n)	a slight, inflamed, pus-filled elevation of the skin	膿皰	脓疱

Notes

English/Chinese Medical Glossary - Q

quadriceps (n)	a large four-part muscle on the front of the leg between the knee and hip	四頭肌	四头肌
Qualified Medicare Beneficiary (QMB) (n)	a person whose income falls below 100% of federal poverty guidelines, for whom the state must pay the Medicare Part B premiums, deductibles, and co-payments	合格的醫療保險受益人	合格的医疗保险受益人
quality of care (n)	the degree or grade of excellence with respect to medical services received by enrollees, administered by providers or programs, in terms of technical competence, needs appropriateness, acceptability, humanity, structure, etc	護理品質	护理质量
quarantine (n)	a period of time during which a vehicle, a person, or material suspected of carrying a contagious disease is detained; enforced isolation imposed to prevent a contagious disease from spreading	檢疫	检疫
queasy (adj)	1. uneasy; 2. having an upset stomach; nauseated; sickening	反胃的	反胃的
quiescent (adj)	marked by a state of inactivity or repose	靜息的	静息的

Notes

English/Chinese Medical Glossary - R

English	Definition	Traditional	Simplified
rabies (n)	an acute, infectious, often fatal viral disease of most warm-blooded animals, esp. wolves, cats, and dogs, that attacks the central nervous system and is transmitted by the bite of the infected animal	狂犬病	狂犬病
radiation (n)	beams of energy used to make x-rays, or to kill cancer cells	放射物	放射物
radioactive (adj)	being capable of releasing radiation	放射性的	放射性的
radioactive iodine (n)	iodine that emits radiation and is used in medical procedures to generate images of the internal structures of the body, usually the thyroid gland	放射性碘	放射性碘
radiography (n)	examining the body with xrays	放射性相術	放射性相术
radiologist (n)	a physician who specializes in the use of ionizing radiation for medical diagnosis, esp. the use of x-rays in medical imaging	放射科醫師	放射科医师
radiology technician (n)	a person trained to maintain and operate x-ray or radiography equipment	放射線技師	放射线技师
radius (n)	the outer, shorter bone of the forearm	橈骨	橈骨
rales, crackles (n)	abnormal sounds during breathing	羅音，肺泡音	罗音，肺泡音
range of motion exercises (n)	a measure of one's flexibility and capabilities in movement, usually examined after an injury	活動度練習	活动度练习
rape (v)	the crime of forcing another person to submit to sexual intercourse	強姦	强奸
rash (n) (m)	a skin eruption	疹	疹
razor (n)	a sharp-edged cutting instrument	剃刀	剃刀
reactive (n)	tending to be responsive or to react to a stimulus	反應的	反应的
reading glasses (n)	glasses worn to assist in focusing while reading	眼鏡	眼镜

English/Chinese Medical Glossary - R

reagent (n)	substance used to detect other substances, used in laboratory testing	試劑	试剂
receptionist (n)	an office worker employed chiefly to receive visitors and answer the telephone	接待員	接待员
recipient (n)	a person who has been designated by a Medicaid agency as eligible to receive Medicaid benefits (sometimes referred to as beneficiary)	接受者	接受者
recommended (v)	endorsed as fit, worthy, or competent	推薦	推荐
reconstitution (n)	the return to an original state of a substance, or combination of parts to make a whole	復原	复原
reconstructive surgery (n)	a surgical procedure that attempts to restore damaged tissue or organs to their original state	整複外科	整复外科
records (n) (m)	medical records; an organized database or file that contains the medical history of one or more patients	醫療記錄	医疗记录
recovery room (n)	a hospital room equipped for the care and observation of patients immediately following surgery	復原室	复原室
rectal (adj)	pertaining to the rectum	直腸的	直肠的
rectum (n)	the distal or end portion of the large intestine, where stool (feces) is stored prior to defecation	直腸	直肠
recuperation (n)	the recovery of health and strength	復原	复原
recurrent (adj)	occurring or appearing again or repeatedly	復發的	复发的
red blood cell (n)	a red-colored cell capable of transporting oxygen throughout the body	紅血球	红血球
reduction (n) (m)	the correction of a fracture, dislocation, or hernia, moving it back to its normal location	復位術	复位术

English/Chinese Medical Glossary - R

reflex (n)	an involuntary action or movement	反射作用	反射作用
reflux (n)	a backward or return flow	回流	回流
refractory (adj)	not responsive to treatment	難治的	难治的
regeneration (n)	the natural renewal of a structure, as of lost tissue or a part	新生	新生
registered nurse (n)	a graduate trained nurse who has passed a state registration examination	註冊護士	注册护士
registration (n)	the act of officially recording items, names, or actions, or the place where such recording is performed	註冊	注册
regression (n)	a return to a former or earlier state	復原	复原
regurgitation (n)	a backward flowing, as the casting up of undigested food, or the backward flowing of blood into the heart, or between the chambers of the heart when a valve is not working properly	回流	回流
rehabilitation (n)	the process of restoring a patient, such as a handicapped person, to optimal life through education and therapy	復原，康復	复原，康复
rehydration (n)	restoration of water or fluid content to a body	再水化	再水化
reinfection (n)	a second infection by the same organism or virus	再感染	再感染
relapse (n)	falling back or reversion to a former state; regression after partial recovery from illness	復發	复发
relative (n)	a person who is related by marriage, ancestry, or family	親屬	亲属
relax (v)	to calm, rest, or reduce mobility; to make loose	鬆弛，放鬆	松弛，放松
relaxant (n)	something, such as a drug or therapeutic treatment, that relaxes or relieves muscular or nervous tension	弛緩的	弛缓的

English/Chinese Medical Glossary - R

relieve (v)	to alleviate or lessen pain or discomfort	減輕	减轻
remedy (n)	something, such as medicine or therapy, that relieves pain, cures disease, or corrects a disorder	藥品	药品
remission (n)	the condition or period when the symptoms of a disease are not visible	減輕	减轻
remove (v)	to take away; to do away with	移除	移除
renal (adj)	pertaining to the kidney	腎臟的	肾脏的
replacement (n)	a substitute	置換	置换
replicate (v)	to duplicate, copy, or repeat	複製	复制
reproductive system (n)	the system of organs, glands, tissues, and hormones involved in reproduction	生殖系統	生殖系统
research (v)	to search or investigate by collecting information	研究	研究
resection (n)	the removal of a portion or all of an organ or other structure	切除術	切除术
resident (n) (m)	a physician serving a period of residency, the period during which a physician receives specialized clinical training	住院醫生	住院医生
respiration (n)	the act or process of inhaling and exhaling; breathing	呼吸	呼吸
respiratory system (n)	the integrated system of organs involved in the intake and exchange of oxygen and carbon dioxide between a human and the atmosphere	呼吸系統	呼吸系统
respite care service (n)	service that provides relief for a patient's caretaker	休息照護服務	休息照护服务
restraints (n)	straps used to restrict movement	約束	约束
resuscitation (n)	the restoration to life or consciousness of one apparently dead	心肺復甦	心肺复苏
retardation (n)	delay, slowness in development or progress	阻滯	阻滞
retina (n)	the inner layer of the eyeball that responds to light and enables sight by sending signals to the brain	視網膜	视网膜

English/Chinese Medical Glossary - R

retinal detachment (n)	a condition where the retina cannot send signals to the brain thereby causing blindness	視網膜脫離	视网膜脱离
retinal disease (n)	a disease of the retina of the eye; the retina is weakened by tiny blood vessels of the eye either from small tears or holes, or lack of blood going to these blood vessels, which results in loss of vision	視網膜疾病	视网膜疾病
retinopathy (n)	a disease or disorder of the retina	視網膜病	视网膜病
retraction (n)	1. act of drawing back; 2. reduction of tissue volume	退縮	退缩
rheumatic fever (n)	a severe infectious disease occurring chiefly in children, characterized by fever and painful inflammation of the joints, and frequently resulting in permanent damage to the valves of the heart	風濕熱	风湿热
rheumatic heart disease (n)	heart disease caused by rheumatic fever	風濕性心臟病	风湿性心脏病
rheumatism (n)	any of several pathological conditions of the muscles, tendons, joints, bones, or nerves, characterized by fever and painful inflammation of the joints	風濕病	风湿病
rheumatoid arthritis (n)	a chronic disease marked by stiffness and inflammation of the joints, weakness, loss of mobility, and deformity	風濕性關節炎	风湿性关节炎
rheumatoid factor test (n)	a test that determines whether a rheumatoid factor is present in the blood; the presence of this factor may indicate rheumatoid arthritis	類風濕性關節炎因數試驗	类风湿性关节炎因子试验
rheumatologist (n)	a physician who studies any of several pathological conditions of the muscles, tendons, joints, bones, or nerves	風濕病學家	风湿病学家

English/Chinese Medical Glossary - R

rhinitis (n)	inflammation of the mucous membrane of the nose	鼻炎	鼻炎
rhinoscope (n)	an instrument used to examine the nasal passages	照鼻鏡	照鼻镜
rhonchus (n)	a snoring sound; a rattling in the throat	鼻音	鼻音
rib (n)	one of a series of long, curved bones, occurring in 12 pairs in human beings and extending from the spine to or toward the sternum or breast plate	肋骨	肋骨
rice (n)	a type of grain (white to brown in color) common in many foods and high in carbohydrates	米	米
rickets (n)	disease marked by bending and distortion of the bones; caused by vitamin D deficiency	軟骨病	软骨病
ring finger (n)	the third finger from the thumb and next to the little finger	無名指	无名指
ringing in the ears (n)	a continuous high pitched noise in the ear, often associated with a history of loud noise exposure	耳鳴	耳鸣
ringworm (n)	any of a number of contagious skin diseases caused by several related fungi, characterized by ring-shaped, scaly, itching patches on the skin	癬	癣
rinse (v)	to wash lightly with water	漱	漱
risk behaviors (n)	activities that may increase the chance of disease or injury	危險行為	危险行为
root canal (n)	a dental procedure that removes an infected part of a tooth	牙根管	牙根管
root of hair (n)	the portion of the hair that connects to the skin and holds the rest of the hair in place	毛根	毛根
rough (adj)	having a bumpy, uneven surface; not smooth or even	粗糙的	粗糙的
rubdown (n)	an energetic massage of the body	按摩	按摩

English/Chinese Medical Glossary - R

rubella (n)	an acute, infectious respiratory and lymphatic system disease; producing a temporary rash; measles	風疹	风疹
runny nose (n)	a condition in which excess mucus is present in the nasal cavity, usually caused by an illness, nasal sinus infection, or allergy	流鼻涕	流鼻涕
rupture (n)	forcible tearing or disruption of tissue; a hernia	破裂	破裂

Notes

English/Chinese Medical Glossary - S

safe sex (n)	sexual intercourse using contraceptive, usually a condom	安全性交	安全性交
safety lock (n)	of, relating to, or containing salt; salty	保險鎖	保险锁
saline (n)	a solution, esp. one that is the same concentration as blood and is used in medicine and surgery	鹽水	盐水
saline abortion (n)	an abortion caused by injecting saline into the womb; used in later stages of pregnancy	鹽析流產	盐析流产
saliva (n)	the watery, tasteless liquid mixture released in the mouth	唾液	唾液
salivary glands (n)	special glands in the mouth that secrete saliva and assist in digestion of food	唾液腺	唾液腺
salivation (n)	the secretion of saliva in the mouth	唾液分泌	唾液分泌
salpingitis (n)	inflammation of the 1. fallopian or 2. Eustachian tubes	輸卵管炎	输卵管炎
salve (n)	a medicinal ointment; something that soothes or heals; balm	軟膏	软膏
sample (n)	a portion, piece, or segment that is representative of a whole	樣本	样本
sanatorium (n)	an institution for the treatment of chronic disease	療養院	疗养院
sanitary napkins (n)	a disposable pad of absorbent material worn to absorb menstrual flow	衛生棉	卫生巾
satisfactory condition (n)	an indication that a patient is doing well and is not in serious danger	病情穩定	病情稳定
scab (n)	the crust-like skin that covers a healing wound	結痂	结痂

English/Chinese Medical Glossary - S

scabies (n)	infestation of the skin by the human itch mite, Sarcaptes; the initial symptom of scabies is the appearance of red, raised bumps that are intensely itchy	疥瘡	疥疮
scald (v)	to burn with or as if with hot liquid or steam	燙	烫
scale (n)	a dry, thin flake of shedding skin	鱗屑	鳞屑
scalp (n)	the skin covering the top of the human head	頭皮	头皮
scaly, dry (adj)	covered or partially covered with scales	鱗狀的，乾燥的	鳞状的，干燥的
scapula (n)	either of two large, flat, triangular bones forming the back part of the shoulder	肩胛骨	肩胛骨
scar (n)	a mark left on the skin following the healing of a surface of an injury or wound	瘢痕	瘢痕
Scarlet Fever (n)	an acute contagious disease occurring predominantly among children and characterized by a red skin eruption and high fever	猩紅熱	猩红热
schizophrenia (n)	a mental disorder which causes severe confusion	精神分裂症	精神分裂症
sciatica (n)	radiating pain from the buttock down the leg	坐骨神經痛	坐骨神经痛
sclera (n)	the white portion of the eye that makes up the outer layer of the eyeball	鞏膜	巩膜
sclerosis (n)	a thickening or hardening of a body part, as of an artery, esp. from tissue hardening, disease, or overgrowth	硬化症	硬化症
scoliosis (n)	abnormal lateral curvature of the spine or back bone	脊柱側凸	脊柱侧凸
scraping (n)	a small piece or bit; fragment	刮除術	刮除术
scratch (v)	1. to make a thin, shallow cut or mark on a surface with a sharp instrument; 2. to rub or scrape the skin to relieve itching	抓傷	抓伤

English/Chinese Medical Glossary - S

screening test (n)	any of various methods use to detect a disease in healthy people	篩選試驗	筛选试验
scrotum (n)	the external sac of skin enclosing the testes	陰囊	阴囊
scrub (surgically) (v)	to rub hard in order to clean	（外科手術上）用力擦洗	（外科手术上）用力擦洗
seafood (n)	any food products that come from the water, including shellfish, sea mammals, and fish	海鮮	海鲜
seat belt (n)	a belt used to secure an individual in his or her seat	安全帶	安全带
sebaceous gland (n)	a gland that secretes oil	皮脂腺	皮脂腺
secondary care (n)	health care necessary to supplement primary care to meet the enrollee's needs, requiring the knowledge of a physician who is a specialist	二級醫療，專科治療	二级医疗，專科治疗
second-hand smoke (n)	environmental tobacco smoke that is inhaled involuntarily or passively by someone who is not smoking; environmental tobacco smoke is generated from the side stream (the burning end) of a cigarette, pipe or cigar or from the exhaled mainstream (the smoke puffed out by smokers) of cigarettes, pipes, and cigars	間接吸煙，二手煙	间接吸烟，二手烟
secrete (v)	to generate and separate out a substance from cells or bodily fluids; to release a fluid or substance	分泌	分泌
secretion (n) (m)	1. the act of generating or separating out a substance from cells or bodily fluids; 2. the result of this process	分泌物	分泌物
sedative (n)	an agent which decreases excitement	鎮靜藥	镇静药
sedentary (adj)	of, or pertaining to a condition of little movement or constant sitting	靜坐的	静坐的

English/Chinese Medical Glossary - S

segment (n)	portion of a larger body or structure	段，節片	段，节片
seizure (n)	a sudden convulsion and involuntary movement of the body	癲癇	癫痫
selectivity (n)	the degree to which a dose of a drug produces a desired effect	選擇性	选择性
semen (n)	a whitish secretion of the male reproductive organs, the transporting medium for spermatozoa or sperm	精液	精液
seminal vesicles (n)	glandular structures that secrete most of the components of semen	精囊	精囊
senility (n)	the physical and mental deterioration associated with old age	衰老	衰老
sensation (n)	a perception associated with stimulation of a sense organ or with a specific bodily condition; the faculty to feel and perceive	感覺	感觉
sense (v)	to become aware of; to perceive	覺	觉
sensitive (adj)	capable of perceiving with a sense or the senses	神經過敏的	神经过敏的
sensory (adj)	of, or pertaining to any organ used to feel, sense, smell, hear, see, or detect any sensation	知覺的	知觉的
septic (adj)	produced by or due to decomposition by microorganisms	膿毒性的	脓毒性的
septicemia (n)	blood poisoning, bacterial infection in the blood	敗血病	败血病
serious condition (n)	a physical or mental condition that could lead to death or considerable damage	病危	病危
seroconversion (n)	the development of detectable specific antibodies as a result of a disease or immunization	血清轉化	血清转化

English/Chinese Medical Glossary - S

English	Definition	Traditional	Simplified
serology (n)	the medical science of studying different fluids to detect the presence of antibodies to specific antigens	血清學	血清学
serum (n)	the clear portion of any body fluid	血清	血清
sex (n)	1. the condition or character of being male or female; the physiological, functional, and psychological differences that distinguish the male and the female; 2. sexual intercourse	①性別；②性欲	①性别；②性欲
sexual relations (n)	an encounter characterized by sexual contact	性關係	性关系
sexually transmitted disease (n)	a contagious disease passed between people during sexual contact	性傳染疾病	性传染疾病
sharp (adj)	any of various instruments that have a thin edge or a fine point, such as a razor or scalpel	鋒利的	锋利的
shin (n)	having a thin edge or a fine point; suitable for or capable of cutting or piercing; a cutting quality as in pain	脛	胫
shinbone (n)	the tibia; the larger bone between the foot and knee	脛骨	胫骨
shingles (n) (m)	a viral infection causing a line of painful blisters along a nerve path	帶狀皰疹	带状疱疹
shiver (v)	to shudder or shake from or as if from cold; to tremble	戰慄，發抖	战栗，发抖
shock (n) (m)	a generally temporary state of massive bodily trauma, usually characterized by marked loss of blood pressure	休克	休克
shock (n) (m)	the sensation and muscular spasm caused by an electric current passing through the body or through a bodily part	肌震顫	肌震颤
shock (v)	to give an electric shock	（使）肌震顫	（使）肌震颤

English/Chinese Medical Glossary - S

shortness of breath (n)	inability to inhale the necessary amount of air; low energy level due to reduced respiratory rate	氣喘；呼吸短促	气喘；呼吸短促
shot (n) (m)	an injection of a drug into a vein, the skin, or muscle	靜脈、皮膚或肌肉注射	静脉、皮肤或肌肉注射
shot (n) (m)	gun shot	槍擊	枪击
shoulder (n)	the part of the human body between the neck and upper arm	肩（部）	肩（部）
shunt (n)	to turn to one side; to divert; to bypass	旁路	旁路
siblings (n)	brother or sister; related to one or both parents	兄弟或姊妹	兄弟或姊妹
side (n)	the left or right half of the trunk of a human	一邊，一面	一边，一面
side effect (n)	a secondary effect, esp. an undesirable secondary effect of a drug or therapy	副作用	副作用
sight (n)	the ability to see	視力	视力
sigmoid colon (n)	the curving end-section of the large intestine	乙狀結腸	乙状结肠
sigmoidoscope (n)	a slender instrument used to examine the area of the colon closest to the anus	乙狀結腸鏡	乙状结肠镜
sign (n) (m)	something that suggests the presence or existence of a fact, condition, or quality, esp. the physical or mental conditions that assist in diagnosing a disease	症狀	症状
simultaneous (adj)	existing or occurring at the same time	同時發生的，同步的	同时发生的，同步的
sinus (n)	a depression or cavity formed by a bending or curving, esp. in the nose or in the heart; air passage behind the nose and face	竇	窦
sinusitis (n)	inflammation of the sinus membrane, esp. in the nasal region	鼻竇炎	鼻窦炎

English/Chinese Medical Glossary - S

skeletal system (n)	the entire collection of bone, connective tissue, and cartilage that supports the body and aids in its movement	骨骼系統，骨系統	骨骼系统，骨系统
skilled nursing facility (n)	a health facility that provides continuous skilled nursing care and supportive care to patients whose primary need is for the availability of 24-hour inpatient care	專業護理設施	专业护理设施
skin (n)	the tissue forming the external covering of the body	皮膚	皮肤
skin test (n)	any of various tests involving pricking the skin to diagnose a disease, esp. tuberculosis	皮膚測試	皮肤测试
skull (n)	the bones of the head that make up the brain case and face	顱骨，頭骨	颅骨，头骨
sleep disorder (n)	any of various conditions that cause difficulties while sleeping	睡眠障礙；失眠	睡眠障碍；失眠
sleep inducing (adj)	of, or pertaining to an agent that causes or forces sleep	催眠的	催眠的
sleep walking (n)	the state of walking or movement on one's feet while still apparently sleeping	夢行症，夢遊	梦行症，梦游
sleeping pills (n)	a sedative, esp. in the form of a pill or capsule, to relieve the inability to sleep	安眠藥	安眠药
sling (n)	a looped rope, strap, or chain for supporting, cradling, or hoisting something, esp. a support for a limb when broken or dislocated	懸帶，吊腕帶	悬带，吊腕带
slipped disk (n)	the abnormal movement of tissue between vertebrae in the backbone	椎間盤突出	椎间盘突出
sliver (n)	a thin piece cut, split, or broken off, esp. a sliver of metal or wood	薄片	薄片
slurred speech (n)	the act of speaking indistinctly by running sounds together	言語不清，言語模糊	言语不清，言语模糊

English/Chinese Medical Glossary - S

small intestine (n)	the part of the intestine, extending from the stomach to the large intestine, in which digestion is completed	小腸	小肠
smell (v)	to perceive the scent of something	嗅，聞	嗅，闻
smoke (v)	to draw in and exhale the smoke of something, such as tobacco	吸煙	吸烟
smoke detector (n)	a fire safety device in a building or home that makes noise in the presence of smoke	煙霧探測器	烟雾探测器
smoking cessation (n)	the act of quitting smoking	戒煙	戒烟
snacks (n)	any prepared food eaten between meals	點心，零食	点心，零食
sneeze (v)	to expel air forcibly from the mouth and nose in an explosive, spasmodic involuntary action	打噴嚏	打喷嚏
sniffles (n)	a condition that prompts someone to sniff repeatedly, as in crying or having a runny nose	抽氣	抽气
snore (v)	to breathe noisily and forcefully through the nose, usually while sleeping	打鼾，打呼嚕	打鼾，打呼噜
soak (v)	to make thoroughly wet or saturated by or as if by placing in liquid	浸；泡；濕透	浸；泡；湿透
soap (n)	a cleansing agent, manufactured in bars, flakes, or liquid form	肥皂	肥皂
Social Security Administration (n)	the agency of Health and Human Services responsible for the social security system	社會安全局	社会安全局
social security number (n)	the number of a particular individual's social security account.	社會安全號碼	社会安全号码

English/Chinese Medical Glossary - S

Social Services Agency (n)	The agency responsible for administering state, federal, and county programs for health care, social services, public assistance, job training, and rehabilitation	社會服務機構	社会服务机构
Social Worker (n)	a professional working within the field of social services	社會工作者	社会工作者
sodium (n)	a metallic element essential for human life and important in muscle activity, found in table salt and in fast foods in high levels	鈉	钠
soft tissue (n)	the tissue including muscle, ligaments, tendons, skin, and fat	軟組織	软组织
sole (n)	the under-surface of the foot	腳掌	脚掌
solid food (n)	food that does not dissolve readily into liquid form; food that requires chewing	固體食物	固体食物
somatic (n)	pertaining to the body or body wall	身體，軀體	身体，躯体
somnolence (n)	sleepiness; unnatural drowsiness	嗜睡	嗜睡
sonogram (n)	ultrasonogram; echogram; image obtained by using ultrasound	超聲波掃描圖	超声波扫描图
sonographer (n)	a technologist trained to use ultrasound equipment	超聲波醫師，超聲波檢測師	超声波医师，超声波检测师
soporific (n)	causing or inducing sleep; also see *sleep inducing* and *sleeping pills*	安眠藥	安眠药
sore (n)	an area painful to touch	傷口，痛處	伤口，痛处
sore throat (n)	any of various inflammations of the tonsils, pharynx, or larynx characterized by pain in swallowing	喉嚨痛	喉咙痛
spasm (n)	a sudden, violent, involuntary contraction of a muscle	痙攣	痉挛
spasmodic (adj)	of, or pertaining to an involuntary movement	痙攣的，間歇性的	痉挛的，间歇性的

English/Chinese Medical Glossary - S

specialist (n)	a doctor who focuses his or her practice of medicine on one organ or area	專科醫生	专科医生
specific (adj)	special, distinctive, or unique, as a quality or attribute	特定的，具體的	特定的，具体的
specimen (n)	an individual, item, or part taken as representative of an entire set or whole; sample	樣品，標本	样品，标本
speculum (n)	1. a mirror or polished metal plate used as a reflector; 2. an instrument for widening the opening of a body cavity for medical examination	①窺鏡；②擴張器	①窥镜；②扩张器
spell (n)	1.a short period of time; 2. an access of disease as in fainting spell	①一段時間；②咒語	①一段时间；②咒语
sperm (n)	spermatozoon; the male contribution to pregnancy	精子	精子
spermicide (n)	an agent that is destructive to sperm	殺精子劑	杀精子剂
sphincter (n) (m)	band of muscles that constrict any passage, as in the stomach or anus	括約肌	括约肌
sphygmomanometer (n)	an instrument used to measure blood pressure; also see *blood pressure cuff*	血壓計	血压计
spinal anesthesia (n)	anesthetic that is injected into the spinal cord	脊椎麻醉	脊椎麻醉
spinal column (n)	the column of bones enclosing the spinal cord; backbone	脊椎	脊椎
spinal cord (n)	the part of the central nervous system contained within the spinal canal and extending from the brain down the back bone	脊髓	脊髓
spine (n)	the combined nerves, cartilage, and bone that comprise the backbone; the columnar assemblage of connecting vertebrae extending from the head to the pelvis, forming the support axis of the body	脊柱	脊柱

English/Chinese Medical Glossary - S

spirometry (n)	a technique of measuring the volume of air entering and leaving the lungs	肺活量測定法	肺活量测定法
spit (n) (m)	saliva, esp. expelled from the mouth	唾液，唾沫	唾液，唾沫
spit (v) (m)	to eject liquid from the mouth	吐唾沫或痰	吐唾沫或痰
spleen (n)	an organ on the left side of the abdomen below the diaphragm that produces white blood cells, filters blood and stores blood cells	脾臟	脾脏
splinter (n)	a sharp, slender piece, as of wood, bone, glass, or metal, split or broken off from the main body	尖片，裂片	尖片，裂片
spores (n)	a microorganism such as bacteria that is easily reproduced and can cause the spread of disease	孢子	孢子
spotting (n)	a slight bloody discharge from the vagina	斑點	斑点
sprain (v)	to cause a painful wrenching of the ligaments of a joint	扭傷	扭伤
sprained (adj)	pertaining to an injury caused by a sprain	扭傷的	扭伤的
spread (v)	to move to other locations within the body	擴散	扩散
sputum (n)	matter ejected through the mouth from the lungs, bronchi, and trachea	痰	痰
squamous (adj)	scaly or platelike; usually referring to tissues of the skin or the lining of tubes	鱗狀的	鳞状的
squeeze (v)	to press together; to compress	擠；壓	挤；压
stab (v)	to pierce or wound with or as if with a pointed object; to plunge a weapon into the body	刺；戳	刺；戳
stable (adj)	of, or pertaining to a physical or mental condition that is not changing	穩定的	稳定的

English/Chinese Medical Glossary - S

stable condition (n)	the medical condition or state of a patient when a disease or injury no longer threatens the patient's life	穩定狀態	稳定状态
standard dosing (n)	an established model of administering medication	標準劑量	标准剂量
standards (n)	authoritative statements of (1) minimum levels of acceptable performance or results, (2) excellent levels of performance or results or (3) the range for acceptable performance or results	標準，規格（其中包括最低標準，最高標準，可接受的範圍）	标准，规格（其中包括最低标准，最高标准，可接受的范围）
stapes (n)	a small bone in the middle ear that assists in hearing	鐙骨	镫骨
stay still (v)	to not move; to relax	靜止不動	静止不动
steady state (n)	a condition of not changing	穩定狀態	稳定状态
sterile (adj)	1. incapable of reproducing sexually; infertile; 2. free of bacteria	①不育的；②消毒的	①不育的；②消毒的
sterility (n)	1. inability to produce offspring; 2. state of being clean and/or free of bacteria	①不孕；②無菌	①不孕；②无菌
sterilization (n)	1. a surgical procedure that prevents someone from reproducing; 2. complete destruction or elimination of all living micro-organisms	①絕育；②消毒，殺菌	①绝育；②消毒，杀菌
sterilize (v)	1. to make someone sterile; 2. to clean an instrument in such a way that it is free of bacteria	①使不育；②殺菌	①使不育；②杀菌
sternum (n)	a long flat bone articulating with the cartilage of and forming the front support for the ribs; breast plate	胸骨	胸骨
steroid (n)	a specific chemical compound involved in proper body function	類固醇	类固醇
stethoscope (n)	an instrument used for listening to sounds produced within the body	聽診器	听诊器
stick out your tongue (v)	to make the tongue visible to a physician for examination	伸出舌頭	伸出舌头

English/Chinese Medical Glossary - S

stiff (adj)	difficult to bend or stretch; rigid	僵硬的	僵硬的
stiffness (n)	the condition of being difficult to bend or stretch	僵硬	僵硬
stillborn (adj)	dead at birth	死產的	死产的
stimulant (n)	something that temporarily arouses or accelerates activity	興奮劑	兴奋剂
stimulate (v)	to excite or make active	刺激	刺激
sting (of an insect) (n)	to pierce or wound painfully with or as if with a sharp-pointed structure or organ, such as that of certain insects	（昆蟲）蜇，叮	（昆虫）蜇，叮
stitches (n)	1. a series of loops of thread through the skin used to hold a wound closed; 2. sharp, stabbing pains	①縫；②刺痛	①缝；②刺痛
stomach (n)	the enlarged, saclike portion of the digestive system between the esophagus and small intestine	胃	胃
stomach ache (n)	pain in the abdomen	胃痛	胃痛
stomach lining (n)	the thick tissue that protects the inside of the stomach	胃粘膜	胃粘膜
stone (n) (m)	mineral matter originating in the kidney, urethra, gallbladder, or bladder	結石	结石
stool (n)	feces; human waste excreted from the anus	糞便	粪便
stool culture (n)	a test used to detect pathogenic organisms in a sample of feces	糞便培養	粪便培养
stool specimen (n)	a sample of feces or bowel movement used to diagnose disease	糞便取樣	粪便取样
strain (v)	to violently stretch or overexert one's muscles	扭傷	扭伤
strained muscle (n)	a muscle damaged by over use or exercise	肌肉拉傷	肌肉拉伤
strengthening (v)	making stronger	鞏固	巩固
strep throat (n)	a specific bacterial infection causing a sore throat	咽喉炎	咽喉炎
stress (n)	forcibly exerted influence; pressure	壓力	压力

English/Chinese Medical Glossary - S

English	Definition	Traditional	Simplified
stress test, exercise treadmill test (n)	a method of evaluating the fitness of a patient, esp. the condition of his/her heart	壓力測試，運動心電圖測試	压力测试，运动心电图测试
stretch (v)	to flex the muscles of the human body	拉伸，伸展	拉伸，伸展
stretcher (n)	a piece of equipment used to transport sick, wounded, or dead people	擔架	担架
stroke (n)	sudden impairment of blood flow to the brain causing paralysis and damage to the brain	中風	中风
stuffy nose (n)	a blocked nasal passage causing difficulties in breathing	鼻塞	鼻塞
stupor (n)	partial or nearly complete unconsciousness	輕度昏迷	輕度昏迷
sty (n)	inflammation of one of the glands in the eyelid	瞼腺炎，麥粒腫	睑腺炎，麦粒肿
subcontract (n)	any agreement entered into by a plan for any services necessary to meet the requirements of their original contract	轉包合同	转包合同
substance abuse (n)	misuse of substances ranging from nicotine (tobacco) and alcohol to other addictive substances such as barbiturates, narcotics, prescription drugs, and the like	濫用藥物	滥用药物
suck (v)	to draw air or liquid into the mouth by inhalation or suction; to draw in by or as if by suction	吸，吸入	吸，吸入
suction curettage (n)	a type of abortion which removes an unborn fetus by using suction	抽吸刮除術	抽吸刮除术
Sudden Infant Death Syndrome (SIDS) (n)	the sudden and unexpected death of a baby with no known illness, typically affecting sleeping infants between the ages of two weeks to six months	嬰兒猝死綜合症	婴儿猝死综合症

English/Chinese Medical Glossary - S

suffer (v)	to feel or sense pain or discomfort	患病，忍受	患病，忍受
suffocate (v)	to impair or prevent respiration; to choke	使窒息	使窒息
suicide (n)	the act or an instance of intentionally killing oneself	自殺	自杀
sunburn (n)	an inflammation or blistering of the skin caused by overexposure to direct sunlight	曬傷	晒伤
sunscreen (n)	a substance in the form of a cream or lotion, used to protect the skin from the damaging ultraviolet rays of the sun	防曬劑	防晒剂
sunstroke (n)	heat stroke caused by exposure to the sun and characterized by a rise in temperature, convulsion, and coma	中暑	中暑
Supplemental Security Income (SSI) (n)	a federally-administered income assistance program authorized by Title XVI of the Social Security Act; SSI provides monthly cash payments in accordance with uniform, nationwide eligibility requirements to needy aged (65 years and older), blind and disabled persons	社會安全補助金	社会安全补助金
support group (n)	a group of people, sometimes led by a therapist, who provide each other moral support, information, and advice on problems relating to some shared characteristic or experience	支援小組	支援小组
suppository (n)	a medicated mass adapted for introduction into the rectal, vaginal, or urethral opening of the body	栓劑	栓剂
surgeon (n)	a physician specializing in surgery	外科醫生	外科医生

English/Chinese Medical Glossary - S

surgery (n)	the treatment of injury, deformity, and disease by instrumental operations	外科手術	外科手术
surgical (adj)	pertaining to or correctable by surgery	外科的	外科的
survey (v)	to query (someone) in order to collect data for the analysis of some aspect of a group or area	調查	调查
swab (n)	a small piece of material attached to the end of a stick or wire and used for obtaining a sample of tissue, for cleaning, or for applying medicine	藥籤	药签
swallow (v)	to cause something, such as food, to pass through the mouth and throat into the stomach	吞咽	吞咽
sweat (n) (m)	perspiration or liquid that is excreted through the pores in the skin	汗水	汗水
sweat (v) (m)	to excrete perspiration or liquid through the pores in the skin	出汗	出汗
sweets (n)	candy; dessert; any of various foods very high in sugar; also see *carbohydrates*	糖果	糖果
swell (v)	to increase in size or volume as a result of internal pressure	膨脹，腫脹	膨胀，肿胀
swelling (n)	something that has increased in volume due to internal pressure	腫脹物	肿胀物
swollen (adj)	of, or pertaining to something that has increased in volume due to internal pressure	腫大的，腫脹的	肿大的，肿胀的
symptom (n)	any subjective evidence of disease or of a patient's condition	症狀	症状
symptomatic (adj)	pertaining to, or of the nature of a symptom	有症狀的	有症状的

English/Chinese Medical Glossary - S

syncope (n)	a loss of consciousness caused by a lack of oxygen to the brain, often caused by a heart condition or low blood pressure	昏厥，暈厥	昏厥，晕厥
syndrome (n)	a set of symptoms which occur together	綜合症	综合症
syphilis (n)	a chronic infectious disease transmitted by direct contact, usually in sexual intercourse	梅毒	梅毒
syringe (n)	a medical instrument used to inject fluids into the body or draw them from it	注射器	注射器
systemic (adj)	of, or pertaining to the entire body	全身的	全身的
systole (n)	a single contraction of the heart; the moment blood is ejected from the heart	心臟收縮	心脏收缩
systolic (adj)	1. of, or pertaining to a contraction of the heart and the moment blood is ejected from the heart; 2. referring to the higher number in a blood pressure reading	收縮的	收缩的

Notes

English/Chinese Medical Glossary - S

English/Chinese Medical Glossary - T

tablet (n)	a small flat pellet of medication to be taken by mouth	藥片	药片
take a deep breath (v)	to inhale as much air as possible; to fill the lungs with air	深呼吸	深呼吸
take off (v)	to remove something, esp. clothing; to undress	脫下	脱下
tampon (n)	a plug of absorbent material inserted into a bodily cavity or wound to stop a flow of blood or absorb secretions, usually used during menstruation	月經棉塞	月经棉塞
tapeworm (n)	any of various ribbon-like, often very long, flatworms that are parasitic and live in the intestines	條蟲	绦虫
taste (n)	the sense that distinguishes the flavor of a substance	味覺	味觉
taste (v)	to distinguish the flavor of a substance	品嘗	品尝
tea spoon (n)	the common small spoon used esp. with tea, coffee, and desserts; a measurement equal to approximately 5 milliliters, (or 5 cc)	茶匙	茶匙
tear (n) (m)	to pull apart or into pieces; to make an opening by ripping; to divide, disunite	眼淚	眼泪
tear (v) (m)	to secrete liquid from around the eye	含淚	含泪
tear (v) (m)	a drop of liquid secreted from around the eye	流淚	流泪
tear duct (n)	a canal or channel from the lachrymal gland that secretes a salty liquid commonly called tears	淚腺	泪腺
technician (n)	an expert in a technique, procedure, or complex task	技師	技师
teenager (n)	a person between the ages of 13 and 19; an adolescent	青少年	青少年
teething (v)	the inflammation when new teeth develop in a baby	出牙，長牙	出牙，长牙

English/Chinese Medical Glossary - T

Telecommunication Device for the Deaf (TDD) (n)	a special type of phone used to communicate with the deaf and hearing impaired	聽障助聽電話	听障助听电话
telephone number (n)	a number assigned to a telephone line for a specific location that is used to call that location	電話號碼	电话号码
temperature (n)	the degree of hotness or coldness of a body or environment	溫度	温度
temple (n) (m)	the flat region on either side of the forehead	廟宇	庙宇
temporary lodging (n)	housing or shelter intended to be used for a limited time	投宿	投宿
tender (adj)	easily bruised; sensitive; painful or sore	敏感的，觸痛的	敏感的，触痛的
tendon (n)	a band of tough, inelastic fibrous tissue that connects a muscle with its bony attachment	肌腱	肌腱
tendonitis (n)	inflammation of tendons and of tendon-muscle attachments	肌腱炎	肌腱炎
tennis elbow, golfer's elbow (n)	tendinitis; inflammation of tendons and of tendon-muscle attachments, usually from overuse	網球肘，高爾夫肘	网球肘，高尔夫肘
tense (adj)	tightly stretched, strained, esp. tense muscles; in a state of mental or nervous tension or stress	緊張的	紧张的
tension (n)	the condition of being stretched or strained, emotional strain or stress	緊張	紧张
terminal (adj)	1. final; ending; the most distant; 2. severity of a medical condition leading to the end of a patient's life	①末端的，終點的；②晚期的	①末端的，终点的；②晚期的
terminally ill (adj)	severity of a patient's medical condition leading to the end of a patient's life	病危	病危
test (n)	a means of examination, trial, or proof, esp. a medical procedure used to diagnosis a disease	檢測，檢查	检测，检查

English/Chinese Medical Glossary - T

test of pulmonary function (n)	any of various medical examinations to assess the function of the lungs and assist in diagnosis of diseases of the lungs; also see *pulmonary function tests (PFT)*	肺功能測試	肺功能测试
test strip (n)	a piece of paper used to determine the acidity of a liquid, or the sugar content of blood	測試條	测试条
test tube (n)	a clear glass tube usually open at one end and rounded at the closed end, used in laboratory experiments	試管	试管
test tube baby (n)	a baby that has been conceived outside the womb through fertilization of an egg removed from the mother	試管嬰兒	试管婴儿
testicle (n)	a testis	睾丸	睾丸
testicular/prostate problems (n)	medical problems involving the male reproductive organs	睾丸炎、前列腺炎	睾丸炎、前列腺炎
testis (n)	the male reproductive gland, normally paired in an external scrotum or sac of skin	睾丸	睾丸
tetanus (n)	an acute, often fatal infectious disease which generally enters the body through wounds	破傷風	破伤风
therapeutic counseling (n)	individual or group counseling to assist with social, psychological, or medical problems	治療性諮詢	治疗性咨询
therapeutics (n)	the art of healing, having healing or curative powers	治療學	治疗学
therapy (n)	treatment of disease	治療	治疗
thermometer (n)	an instrument for measuring temperature	溫度計	温度计
thigh (n)	the portion of the human leg between the hip and the knee; femur	大腿	大腿
thighbone (n)	the femur; the large bone between the knee and hip	大腿骨	大腿骨
thoracic (adj)	pertaining to or affecting the chest	胸的，胸廓的	胸的，胸廓的

English/Chinese Medical Glossary - T

thorax (n)	the chest and the organs and tissue within it, including the heart, lungs, esophagus, and ribs	胸，胸腔	胸，胸腔
throat (n)	the portion of the digestive tract that lies between the rear of the mouth and the esophagus	咽喉	咽喉
throat drops, lozenges (n)	medication administered directly into the throat in drop form or as a candy, used to decrease the irritation of a sore throat	喉糖，含片	喉糖，含片
throb (v)	to vibrate, pulsate, or sound rapidly or violently with steady rhythm; to pound	悸動	悸动
throbbing (adj)	of, or pertaining to something that throbs, esp. in reference to a headache or injury	悸動的	悸动的
thrombophlebitis (n)	inflammation of a vein caused by a blood clot	血栓性靜脈炎	血栓性静脉炎
thrombosis (n)	the formation, presence, or development of a blood clot in a blood vessel	血栓形成	血栓形成
thrombus (n)	a blood clot blocking a blood vessel or formed in a heart cavity	血栓	血栓
thrush (n)	a yeast infection causing white spots in the mouth	鵝口瘡	鹅口疮
thumb (n)	the short first digit of the human hand, opposable to each of the other four digits	拇指	拇指
thyroid (n)	a two-lobed gland that produces hormones, located in front of and on either side of the throat in humans	甲狀腺	甲狀腺
thyroid problems (n)	problems related to the thyroid	甲狀腺病	甲狀腺病
thyroid stimulating hormone (n)	thyrotropin; a hormone that stimulates or promotes activity of the thyroid gland and regulates body weight; an elevated thyroid stimulating hormone indicates a low thyroid level	甲狀腺刺激素	甲狀腺刺激素

English/Chinese Medical Glossary - T

thyroid stimulating hormone assay (n)	a test to determine the level of thyroid stimulating hormone in the body	促甲狀腺激素測定	促甲状腺激素测定
thyroid test (n)	a procedure used to determine the level of hormones released by the thyroid and to assist in diagnosis	甲狀腺測試	甲状腺测试
tibia (n)	the larger of two bones between the knee and ankle	脛骨	胫骨
tick (insect) (n)	any of numerous bloodsucking parasites that transmit infectious diseases	扁虱（昆蟲）	扁虱（昆虫）
tie the tubes (v)	a surgical procedure that renders a female infertile or unable to become pregnant	結紮輸卵管	结扎输卵管
tight (adj)	cramped; constrained; constricted; snug, often uncomfortably so	緊的	紧的
tightness (n)	the condition of being tight	發緊	发紧
tinea, ringworm (n)	any of various fungous skin diseases	癬	癣
tingling (adj)	of, or pertaining to a prickling, stinging sensation, as from cold, a sharp slap, or excitement	麻，痛感	麻，痛感
tiredness (n)	the condition of being worn-out or fatigued	疲倦	疲倦
tissue (n)	a collection of cells that share a similar function, the soft parts of the body	組織	组织
toddler (n)	a young child between the ages of about one and three years learning to walk	幼兒	幼儿
toe (n)	one of the digits of the foot	腳趾	脚趾
toenail (n)	the hard covering on a toe	腳趾甲	脚趾甲
tolerance (n)	the ability to endure unusually large doses of a drug or toxin	耐藥性	耐药性
tongue (n)	the fleshy muscular organ, attached to the floor of the mouth, that is the principle organ of taste, an important organ of speech, and that aids chewing and swallowing	舌頭	舌头

English/Chinese Medical Glossary - T

tonometry (n)	the diagnostic procedure that uses an instrument to measure the pressure within the eyeball	眼壓測量	眼压测量
tonsillectomy (n)	surgical removal of the tonsils	扁桃腺切除術	扁桃腺切除术
tonsillitis (n)	inflammation of the tonsils	扁桃體炎	扁桃体炎
tonsil (n)	a mass of tissue, esp. either of two such masses, embedded in the walls between the mouth and pharynx	扁桃體	扁桃体
tooth (n)	one of a set of hard, bone-like structures rooted in sockets in the jaws	牙齒	牙齿
tooth brush (n)	a brush used for cleaning teeth	牙刷	牙刷
tooth decay (n)	the destruction or decomposition of a tooth, usually caused by disease	蛀牙，齲齒	蛀牙，龋齿
tooth socket (n)	a hollow cavity in which the roots of a tooth are held in place	牙槽	牙槽
toothache (n)	an aching pain in or near a tooth	牙痛	牙痛
toothpaste (n)	a paste for cleaning teeth	牙膏	牙膏
topic (n)	a subject or theme of a discussion or conversation	主題	主题
topical (adj)	pertaining to a particular surface area; of, or applied to an isolated part of the body; something applied to the skin	局部的，表面的	局部的，表面的
torn (adj)	of, or pertaining to something that has been pulled apart or into pieces, divided, esp. a ligament	破碎的，撕碎的	破碎的，撕碎的
torsion (n)	a type of mechanical stress where an object is twisted and contorted	扭力	扭力
torso (n)	the trunk of the human body	軀幹	躯干
total knee	a surgical procedure that removes a section of the bone around the knee and replaces it with an artificial joint	全膝	全膝

English/Chinese Medical Glossary - T

touch (v)	to feel; to come in contact with something by using a hand or finger	觸摸	触摸
tourniquet (n)	a device used to temporarily stop the flow of blood through a large artery in a limb	止血帶	止血带
towel (n)	a piece of cloth used for drying or cleaning	毛巾	毛巾
toxemia (n)	condition resulting from the spread of bacterial products in the bloodstream; high blood pressure and seizures caused by pregnancy	毒血症	毒血症
toxic (adj)	pertaining to the nature of poison; harmful, destructive, or deadly	有毒的	有毒的
toxicity (n)	quality of being poisonous	毒性	毒性
toxin (n)	a poison	毒素	毒素
trachea (n)	a thin-walled tube of cartilage and membrane tissue descending from the larynx to the bronchi and carrying air to the lungs	氣管	气管
tracheitis (n)	inflammation of the trachea	氣管炎	气管炎
tracheotomy (n)	the act or procedure of cutting into the trachea through the neck to provide an air passage	氣管切開術	气管切开术
traction (n)	the act of drawing or pulling	牽引力	牵引力
traditional healer (n)	competent to provide health care by using vegetable, animal and mineral substances and certain other methods based on the social, cultural and religious background as well as on the knowledge, attitudes and beliefs that are prevalent in the community regarding physical, mental and social well-being and the causation of disease and disability (The Promotion and Development of Traditional Medicine - TRS 622, WHO, Geneva, 1978)	傳統醫療師	传统医疗师

English/Chinese Medical Glossary - T

trainee (n)	student; resident; a person learning a specific field, technique, or skill	實習生	实习生
tranquilize (v)	to calm or reduce mental activity, usually by administering a medication	（使）安靜，（使）鎮靜	（使）安静，（使）镇静
tranquilizer (n)	a drug with a calming, soothing effect	鎮靜劑	镇静剂
transdermal (adj)	entering through the skin	經過皮膚的	经过皮肤的
transfusion (n)	introduction of whole blood directly into the blood stream	輸血	输血
translator (n)	a person who translates written texts	翻譯	翻译
transplant procedure (n)	an operation in which tissue or an organ is transplanted from one person (the donor) to another (the recipient)	移植手術	移植手术
transplantation (n)	the transfer of tissue or an organ from one body, or body part, to another	移植	移植
transportation/escort	assistance for clients who require personal care or support while being transported	運輸、護送	运输、护送
transportation/regular (n)	assist client to transit to a designated place	運輸，定期	运输，定期
transverse colon (n)	the middle section of the large intestine	橫結腸	横结肠
trauma (n)	a wound, esp. one produced by sudden physical injury	外傷	外伤
traumatic (adj)	relating to or resulting from trauma	創傷的	创伤的
treatment (n)	the use or application of remedies with the goal of effecting a cure; therapy	治療，療法	治疗，疗法
tremor (n)	an involuntary trembling or quivering	顫抖	颤抖
triggers (n)	allergens such as pollen, dust, or animal dander that cause an asthma episode (attack)	刺激物	刺激物
tubal ligation (n)	female sterilization; surgical procedure that prevents a woman from reproducing	輸卵管結紮	输卵管结扎

English/Chinese Medical Glossary - T

tube (n)	a hollow cylinder, esp. one that conveys a fluid or functions as a passage; any of various tubes or tube-like structures in the human body including the fallopian tubes, the Eustachian tubes, the urethra, and ureter	管	管
tuberculine test (n)	any of various tests used to determine past or present infection with a bacteria called tubercle bacillus	結核菌素測試	结核菌素测试
tuberculosis (n)	a contagious disease that damages bone, the lungs, and other parts of the body	肺結核	肺结核
tuberculostatic (adj)	inhibiting the growth of tuberculosis	抗結核的	抗结核的
tumor (n)	an abnormal tissue growth	腫瘤	肿瘤
tunnel vision (n)	a reduced field of vision in which vision is limited to the center; extreme narrow view	管狀視力	管状视力
turn over (v)	to move or rotate the entire body in one direction to reveal the back or front side	翻轉	翻转
tweezers (n)	a small, usually metal, tool used for handling small objects	鑷子	镊子
twins (n)	two offspring produced in the same pregnancy	孿生，雙胞胎	孪生，双胞胎
twitch (n)	a sudden small involuntary movement; jerk	抽搐	抽搐
tympanic membrane (n)	ear drum; a thin membrane that divides the outer ear from the middle ear	骨膜	骨膜
typhoid fever (n)	an acute, highly infectious disease transmitted by contaminated food or water and characterized by red rashes, high fever, and intestinal bleeding	傷寒症	伤寒症

Notes

English/Chinese Medical Glossary - T

English/Chinese Medical Glossary - U

ulcer (n)	a local defect of the surface of an organ or tissue; an inflammatory cut on the skin or internal surface of the body, often refers to a painful defect in the stomach lining	潰瘍	溃疡
ulceration (n)	formation or development of an ulcer	潰瘍	溃疡
ulna (n)	the bone extending from the elbow to the wrist on the side opposite the thumb	尺骨	尺骨
ultrasound (n)	high frequency sound used in diagnostic imaging of internal organs	超聲波	超声波
Ultraviolet (UV) Protection (n)	protection from the UV radiation of the sun	紫外線防護	紫外线防护
ultraviolet treatment (n)	therapy used to treat psoriasis, a disease causing lesions on the skin, by using ultraviolet radiation	紫外線療法	紫外线疗法
umbilical cord (n)	the flexible, cord-like structure connecting the unborn baby to the mother at the navel; it supplies blood to the baby and removes the baby's waste	臍帶	脐带
unconscious (adj)	without conscious awareness, asleep and unable to respond to sensory stimuli	無意識的	无意识的
underarm (n)	armpit	腋下	腋下
undernourished (adj)	the condition of being provided insufficient quantity and quality of food to sustain proper health and growth	營養不良的	营养不良的
uniform (n)	marked by lack of variation	制服	制服
unilateral (adj)	affecting only one side, esp. one half of the body	單側的	單側的
unsafe (adj)	harmful or dangerous	危險的	危险的
unwanted (adj)	not wanted, required, or needed	不需要的，多餘的	不需要的，多余的
upper (adj)	higher in place, position, or rank	上面	上面

English/Chinese Medical Glossary - U

upper arm (n)	the section of the arm between the shoulder and elbow	上臂	上臂
upper respiratory infection (n)	any of various infections of the bronchi, nasal passages, throat, or sinus passages	上呼吸道感染	上呼吸道感染
upset stomach (n)	a condition where the stomach is disturbed, not functioning normally, and agitated	腸胃不適	肠胃不适
ureter (n)	the tube that carries fluid from the kidney to the bladder	輸尿管	输尿管
urethra (n)	the canal through which urine is discharged from the bladder	尿道	尿道
urethroscope (n)	a slender instrument used to visually examine the interior of the urethra	尿道鏡	尿道镜
urgency (n)	the sudden compelling urge or need to take action, esp. to urinate	緊急	紧急
urgent care (n)	services required to prevent serious deterioration of health following the onset of an unforeseen condition or injury (i.e., sore throats, fever, lacerations, and broken bones)	適時治療	适时治疗
uric acid (n)	a product of metabolism found in blood and urine; also see *gout*	尿酸	尿酸
urinalysis (n)	the chemical analysis or examination of urine	驗尿	验尿
urinary (adj)	pertaining to the urine; containing or secreting urine	泌尿的	泌尿的
urinary system (n)	the system of organs, tissues, and functions that are involved in urination or the excretion of urine	泌尿系統	泌尿系统
urinary tract infection (n)	an infection of the urinary tract with microorganisms	尿道感染	尿路感染
urinate (v)	to excrete urine; to discharge water and waste from the bladder	小便	小便

English/Chinese Medical Glossary - U

urination (n)	the act of discharging water and waste from the bladder	排尿	排尿
urine (n)	the fluid and dissolved substances secreted by the kidneys, stored in the bladder, and excreted from the body through the urethra	尿	尿
urogenital (adj)	pertaining to the urinary and genital apparatus	泌尿生殖器的	泌尿生殖器的
urologist (n)	the physician who specializes in the physiology and pathology of the genitourinary tract	泌尿科醫師	泌尿科医师
uterine lining (n)	the tissue that lines the inside of the uterus which is lost during menstruation	子宮內膜	子宮内膜
uterus (n)	hollow muscular female organ that holds a developing fetus	子宮	子宮
utilization (n)	the rate patterns of service usage or types of service occurring within a specified time.	利用率	利用率
utilization (n)	the usage of something	利用	利用
uvula (n)	the small, fleshy mass of tissue suspended from the roof of the mouth above the back of the tongue	小舌	小舌

Notes

English/Chinese Medical Glossary - V

vaccinate (v)	to administer a vaccine in order to prevent a future disease from developing	接種疫苗	接种疫苗
vaccination (n)	introduction of vaccine into the body for the purpose of inducing immunity	接種疫苗	接种疫苗
vaccine (n)	a suspension of a killed microorganism or other substance, injected into the body as prevention against a disease	疫苗	疫苗
vagina (n)	the passage leading from the uterus to the external female genitalia	陰道	阴道
vaginal (adj)	pertaining to the vagina	陰道的	阴道的
vaginal bleeding (n)	bleeding through the vagina during menstruation, pregnancy, miscarriage, abortion, or tumor	陰道出血	阴道出血
vaginal yeast infection (n)	a fungus infection of the vagina that causes irritation	陰道酵母菌感染	阴道酵母菌感染
vaginitis (n)	inflammation of the vagina	陰道炎	阴道炎
valve (n) (m)	a membranous structure in a hollow organ or a passage, as in an artery or a vein, that retards or prevents the return flow of a bodily fluid	瓣膜	瓣膜
varicose vein (n)	an abnormal swelling of a vein of the leg	靜脈曲張	静脉曲张
vascular (adj)	of, pertaining to, characterized by, or containing vessels for the transmission or circulation of fluids, esp. blood	血管的	血管的
vasculitis (n)	inflammation of a vessel	血管炎	血管炎
vasectomy, male sterilization (n)	surgical procedure that makes a male infertile	輸精管切除，男性絕育術	输精管切除，男性绝育术

English/Chinese Medical Glossary - V

vegetative state (n)	coma; a state of involuntary or unconscious functioning, esp. after severe head trauma or brain disease, in which an individual is incapable of voluntary or purposeful acts, and is thought to be unable to think or feel	植物人狀態	植物人状态
vein (n)	a vessel that transports blood toward the heart	靜脈	静脉
vena cava (n)	the large vein in the body that brings blood from the body to the heart	腔靜脈	腔静脉
venereal (adj)	pertaining or related to, or transmitted by sexual contact	性病的	性病的
venereal disease (n)	a disease that is transmitted by sexual contact; sexually transmitted disease	性病	性病
venous (adj)	of, or pertaining to the veins	靜脈的	静脉的
ventilator (n)	breathing machine; an instrument that assists someone's respiration, ensuring that an adequate amount of oxygen reaches the lungs	呼吸機	呼吸机
ventricle (n)	either of two muscular chambers of the heart that are responsible for forcing blood away from the heart	心室	心室
vertebra (n)	any of the bone segments forming the spinal column or back bone	脊椎骨	脊椎骨
vertigo (n)	the sensation of dizziness and the feeling that oneself or one's environment is whirling about	眩暈	眩晕
viral (adj)	pertaining to the nature of virus or symptoms of a virus, esp. in characterizing an infection	病毒的	病毒的
Viral Hepatitis (n)	liver infection caused by a virus	病毒性肝炎	病毒性肝炎

English/Chinese Medical Glossary - V

English	Definition	Traditional	Simplified
viral illness (n)	any of various diseases caused by organisms smaller than can be seen with a microscope	病毒性疾病	病毒性疾病
virus (n)	any of various disease-causing organisms, smaller than can be seen with a microscope, that can enter and reproduce in a cell	病毒	病毒
vision (n)	the act or faculty of seeing; sight	視力	视力
visiting nurse (n)	a nurse that provides health care in the home or outside of a hospital or clinic	家庭病房護士	家庭病房护士
visual fields examination (n)	a procedure used to determine a patient's range of sight or vision, to see if all parts of the eye are seeing properly	視野檢查	视野检查
vital capacity (n)	the volume of gas that can be expelled from the lungs after a deep breath	肺活量	肺活量
vitamin (n)	any of various relatively complex substances occurring naturally in plant and animal tissue and essential in small amounts for human metabolism and function	維生素	维生素
vitamin supplements (n)	oral medication used to supply the body with essential vitamins that might be at low levels in the body	維生素補充劑	维生素补充剂
vitreous humor (n)	the clear fluid inside the eyeball	玻璃狀液	玻璃状液
vocal cord (n)	the lower of two pairs of bands or folds in the larynx that vibrate when pulled together and when air is passed up from the lungs, producing sounds and voice	聲帶	声带
voice box (n)	the larynx and vocal cords, organs that enable speech	喉頭	喉头
vomit (n)	matter ejected from the stomach through the mouth	嘔吐	呕吐

English/Chinese Medical Glossary - V

vomit (v)	to eject part or all of the contents of the stomach through the mouth, usually in a series of involuntary muscle contractions	嘔吐	呕吐
vulva (n)	the external female genitalia	外陰	外阴
vulvovaginitis (n)	inflammation of the vulva and vagina; vaginitis	外陰陰道炎	外阴阴道炎

Notes

English/Chinese Medical Glossary - W

waist (n)	the part of the human trunk between the bottom of the rib cage and the pelvis	腰	腰
waiting room (n)	a place where people can sit and rest while waiting, as in a doctor's office	候診室	候诊室
walker (n)	a frame device used to support a person while walking	助行器	助行器
warm-up (v)	a low-intensity aerobic exercise that involves stretching for 5-10 minutes to prevent muscle and skeletal injuries	熱身	热身
wart (n)	a small, circular, hard growth on the hands or feet caused by a virus	瘊子	瘊子
watery eyes (n)	a condition where the lens of the eye is covered with excess fluid secreted from the lachrymal gland, usually caused by an allergic reaction or irritation	流淚眼	流泪眼
weak (adj)	lacking physical strength, energy, or vigor; likely to fail under pressure, stress, or strain	虛弱	虚弱
weak spot (n)	a location or area that has the quality or is in a state of weakness	薄弱點	薄弱点
weakness (n)	the condition of being weak	弱點	弱点
wean (v)	to withhold mother's milk from the young and substitute other food; to slowly reduce a treatment	斷奶；戒掉	断奶；戒掉
weight (over, under, gain, lose) (n)	a measurement of heaviness or mass of a person	重量（超重、體重過輕、增肥、減肥）	重量（超重、体重过轻、增肥、减肥）
weight management (n)	a program based on eating a balanced diet, getting regular exercise, and learning to feel good about your body	體重控制	体重控制

English/Chinese Medical Glossary - W

welfare (n)	the provision of economic or social benefits to a certain group of people, esp. aid furnished by the government or by private agencies to the needy or disabled	福利	福利
well care visit schedule (n)	a schedule of well-care visits for children as recommended by the American Academy of Pediatrics (AAP)	健康護理計劃	健康护理计划
wet the bed (v)	to urinate unknowingly or involuntarily while sleeping	尿床	尿床
wheals (n)	an acute swelling or thickening of the skin	風疹塊	风疹块
wheelchair (n)	a chair mounted on large wheels used to assist a person who is sick, disabled, or incapable of walking	輪椅	轮椅
wheeze (v)	to breathe with difficulty, producing a hoarse whistling sound	喘息	喘息
white blood cells (n)	cells found in the blood that are responsible for fighting infection and disease; leukocytes	白血球	白血球
whooping cough (n)	an infectious disease involving the respiratory passages and characterized by spasms of coughing with deep, noisy inspiration; pertussis	百日咳	百日咳
WIC (Special Supplemental Nutrition Program for Women, Infants & Children) (n)	health care referrals, and nutrition education to pregnant women, new mothers, and their infants	婦女、嬰兒及兒童特別補充營養計劃	妇女、婴儿及儿童特别补充营养计划
windpipe (n)	airway; trachea; the passage through which air reaches the lungs	氣管	气管
wisdom tooth (n)	one of four molars, the last teeth on each side of both jaws, usually appearing later than other teeth	智齒	智齿

English/Chinese Medical Glossary - W

withdrawal (n)	1. the act or process of removing or taking away; 2. symptoms experienced when an addictive substance is stopped	①撤銷；②戒毒過程中出現的症狀	①撤销；②戒毒过程中出现的症状
womb (n)	the uterus; a hollow muscular female organ that holds a developing fetus	子宮	子宫
work related injury (n)	an injury caused by or occurring at work	工傷	工伤
work release (n)	documentation provided by a doctor that states the patient is capable of performing specific work	回復工作證明	回復工作證明
World Health Organization (WHO) (n)	a United Nations agency that coordinates international health activities and helps governments improve health services	世界衛生組織	世界卫生组织
worry (v)	to feel uneasy about; to be troubled	擔心，憂慮	担心，忧虑
wound (n)	an injury, esp. one in which the skin is torn, pierced, cut, or otherwise broken	創傷	创伤
wrist (n)	the junction between the hand and forearm	腕，腕關節	腕，腕关节

Notes

English/Chinese Medical Glossary - XYZ

x-ray (n) (m)	a photograph created by x-ray imaging of bone and internal organs	X射線	X射线
x-ray (v) (m)	to photograph with x-rays used in diagnostic imaging of bone and internal organs	X光檢測	X光检测
yawn (n)	a large inhalation of air while holding the mouth wide open, esp. when tired or needing sleep	哈欠	哈欠
yeast (n)	any of various single-cell fungi that reproduce by budding and are capable of fermenting sugars	酵母	酵母
yeast infection (n)	infection caused by yeast	酵母菌感染	酵母菌感染
yellow fever (n)	an acute infectious disease transmitted by mosquitos, causing vomiting and yellow coloring of the skin	黃熱病	黄热病
zinc (n)	a mineral essential for proper body function	鋅	锌

Notes

English/Chinese Medical Glossary – Reference Sheet

Reference Pages

The Medical Team

Term	Traditional	Simplified
Advanced Registered Nurse Practitioner (ANRP)	高級註冊執業護士	高级注册执业护士
Anesthetist	麻醉師	麻醉师
Attending Physician	主治醫生	主治医生
Certified Nurse Midwife	註冊助產護士	注册助产护士
Counselor	顧問	顾问
Doctor	醫生	医生
Family Doctor	家庭醫生	家庭医生
Licensed Practical Nurse (LPN)	持證執業護士	持证执业护士
Nutritionist	營養學家	营养学家
Pediatrician	兒科醫師	儿科医师
Pharmacist	藥劑師	药剂师
Physical Therapist	理療師	理疗师
Psychiatrist	精神病學家	精神病学家
Psychologist	心理學家	心理学家
Receptionist	接待員	接待员
Registered Nurse (RN)	註冊護士	注册护士
Social Worker	社會工作者	社会工作者
Surgeon	外科醫生	外科医生
Visiting Nurse	外科醫生	外科医生

English/Chinese Medical Glossary - Reference Sheet

Medical Specialists

Term	Traditional	Simplified
Cardiologist	心臟病學家	心脏病学家
Dermatologist	皮膚科醫生	皮肤科医生
Endocrinologist	內分泌學家	内分泌学家
Gastroenterologist	胃腸病醫生	胃肠病医生
Gynecologist	婦科學家	妇科学家
Obstetric Nurse	助產師	助产士
Obstetrician	產科醫師	产科医师
Ophthalmologist	眼科醫師	眼科医师
Optometrist	驗光師	验光师
Orthodontist	矯形齒科醫師	矫形齿科医师
Orthopedist	骨科矯形醫師	骨科矫形医师
Pathologist	病理學家	病理学家
Pulmonologist	肺臟學家	肺脏学家
Radiologist	放射科醫師	放射科医师

English/Chinese Medical Glossary - Reference Sheet

Medical Procedures and Exams

Term	Traditional	Simplified
Biopsy	活組織檢查	活组织检查
Blood Test	驗血	验血
Bone Scan	骨骸掃描	骨骸扫描
Catheterization	心導管術	心导管术
Colonoscopy	結腸鏡檢查	结肠镜检查
Computer Topography Scan	電腦掃描	电脑扫描
Electrocardiogram	心電圖	心电图
Electroencephalography	腦電描記法	脑电描记法
Injection	注射	注射
Lumbar Puncture, Spinal Tap	腰椎穿刺，脊椎穿刺	腰椎穿刺，脊椎穿刺
Magnetic Resonance Imaging	核磁共振	核磁共振
Needle Aspiration Biopsy	針吸活檢	针吸活检
Operation	手術	手术
Surgery	外科手術	外科手术
Ultrasound	超聲波	超声波
X-Ray	X射線	X射线

English/Chinese Medical Glossary - Reference Sheet

Types of Pain

Term	Traditional	Simplified
Ache	隱﹞痛	隐﹞痛
Burning Pain	灼痛	灼痛
Constant Pain	疼痛持續	疼痛持续
Cramp	痛性痙攣	痛性痉挛
Dull Pain	隱痛	隐痛
On and Off Pain	陣痛	阵痛
Pain	疼痛	疼痛
Radiating Pain	疼痛擴散	疼痛扩散
Sharp Pain	銳痛	锐痛
Shooting Pain	刺痛	刺痛
Throbbing Pain	抽痛	抽痛

English/Chinese Medical Glossary - Reference Sheet

Medical Equipment

Term	Traditional	Simplified
Bandage	繃帶	绷带
Bedpan	便盆	便盆
Blood Pressure Cuff	血壓表袖套	血压表袖套
Brace	支持〔保護〕支架	支持（保護）支架
Cast (Plaster)	石(膏)	石(膏)
Catheter	導管	导管
Forceps	鉗子	钳子
Gauze	紗布	纱布
Monitor	監視器	监视器
Needle, Syringe	注射針	注射针
Otoscope	耳鏡	耳镜
Rhinoscope	照鼻鏡	照鼻镜
Speculum	①窺鏡；②擴張器	①窥镜；②扩张器
Stethoscope	聽診器	听诊器
Ventilator	呼吸機	呼吸机

Made in the USA
Coppell, TX
05 October 2024